RONALD WILSON

101 Things

Your Barber/

Stylist Hates

(But May Never Tell You)

WESTBOW·
PRESS
A DIVISION OF THOMAS NELSON
& ZONDERVAN

Scripture taken from the King James Version of the Bible.

WestBow Press books may be ordered through booksellers or by contacting:

WestBow Press
A Division of Thomas Nelson & Zondervan
1663 Liberty Drive
Bloomington, IN 47403
www.westbowpress.com
1 (866) 928-1240

ISBN: 978-1-4908-8571-1 (sc)
ISBN: 978-1-4908-8573-5 (hc)
ISBN: 978-1-4908-8572-8 (e)

Library of Congress Control Number: 2015910082

Print information available on the last page.

WestBow Press rev. date: 06/26/2015

ACKNOWLEDGEMENTS

I must start by acknowledging my wife, Rachel for sacrificing and allowing me the countless hours it took me to accomplish this project. You understood my heart concerning this writing and allowed me the space to complete this assignment to barbers and stylists across the country. You knew how much finishing this writing meant to me and you didn't allow me to give up. In the seasons I almost gave up on this writing, you were always there to push me and inspire me to finish. There are not enough words I can write to thank you for your prayers and support. May God richly bless you and all that you put your hands to do! I'm overjoyed and will be forever grateful for God giving me you!

To my sons Ronald and Gabriel, I thank God for you every day and I'm forever grateful that God saw fit and trusted me to father you. Every time I look at you I receive a fresh breath of air that empowers me with the strength and courage I need to press on. You will never begin to imagine the major role you played in keeping me focused while tackling this assignment. You also sacrificed family time and although you may have not understood, you yet allowed me the time I was in need of to write. To my son Day'quan and my daughter Ty'kia, I love you and thank God for placing you in my life. Thank you for being understanding. Through it all you have loved me regardless. I thank you both for believing in me. To my mother Mae, who raised me up the best she could while facing the challenges of being a single parent while battling poverty. You taught me how to survive and provide even when the pressures of life are present at times. You are the greatest mother a child could ever have. I love you mom!

I'm grateful to the body of Kingdom Vision Life Center in Greensboro, NC. Thank you for your prayers. I thank you for believing in the God in me and allowing me to speak into your lives on a day to day basis. May God continue to bless you with life and favor.

To my spiritual father the late Bishop John W. Barber. I thank God for the many times you laid your hands upon me and spoke into my life. You stained my spirit with a deep hunger for God and you taught me by example how to believe God through tough times. Words will never be able to express the life changing impression God transferred and imparted into me through your life! To my spiritual father and mentor Bishop Michael Blue. You are a walking inspiration to me and your life constantly encourages and challenges me to walk in a spirit of excellence! Every time you open your mouth my life is transformed! Thank you sir.

Finally the greatest thanks of ALL belong to the Bishop of my soul, my saviour and King, the Lord Jesus Christ. I am forever grateful for you gracing me with the years you have allowed me to walk along your side. Without God giving me the drive and the passion, none of this writing would have been possible. Thank you for the wisdom and the ability to birth out the seed that was planted into my spirit concerning this project. Praise God from whom all blessings flow. Everything that happened to me that was good, *God did it!*

CONTENTS

DEDICATION

This book is dedicated to every barber and stylist in America and beyond. I thank you for your longsuffering and willingness to dedicate your life behind your barber's chair to help groom the world at large. It's you that keep the world looking good. From taking family pictures to going on a date, to going in for an interview, barbers have dedicated their lives to help those endeavors to go a lot smoother. Rather your customer was on a first date, a fifty year anniversary date or traveling overseas on a corporate business trip, you were there with him or her in the presence of a haircut. I remember telling one of my customers that was traveling to New York for a business trip that I would be there with him. He didn't understand at first but after I explained to him that wherever he goes I'm there with him because of the haircut he was wearing. Afterwards we both laughed as he agreed to the statement.

Again, thanks for your commitment and loyalty

to the community. You are literally responsible for landing people jobs, relationships, great photo shots and much more. I cannot imagine what this world would be like without a barber or a stylist. Thanks for putting up with all the things that comes your way at the shop. You stood in there and because of your stand the world is a more beautiful place! Literally!

INTRODUCTION

This book is written to guide every customer on a personal, virtual tour, through the head of barbers and hairstylists across the globe. From North Carolina, to the coasts of sunny California, barbers and stylists are often blamed for everything under the sun as pertaining to cutting and styling the hair of public America. Things such as, pushing a customer' s hair line back, missing appointments that were not made, drying out a customer' s scalp, giving someone's child a ringworm, making someone's hair fall out or thin out, even down to "you are the reason I'm bald!" The list carries on, but I will spare myself the time to get down to other areas that need to be discussed.

I will admit that some barbers and stylists do foolish things at times. Things such as walking away from customers to chat on their cell phones. This is done after seating the customer and putting the cape on him or her. Some barbers cut off their clippers while cutting hair to add to a joke, and even instigate at times to get something started that wasn't there. The truth of the matter is if every customer knew what their barber had to put up with on a day to day basis while cutting hair everyday for eight to twelve hours a day, they will be amazed they still have a barber. Although I'm sure there are many more, I only had the time to bring into the light 101 things that are in constant rotation that our loyal customer's do, that we as barbers and stylists hate but may never tell you! I know hate is a strong word but if you stood in the shoes of your barber or stylist, you may feel me a little more.

Growing up, for me, a trip to the neighborhood barbershop was never anticipated. I remember my mom, and my aunt taking me to get my first haircut. I remember walking into a stare from total strangers. My world froze and everything seemed as though it shifted into slow motion. A group of older men were looking and pointing in our direction. "Get me out of here" was the only thought that came to my mind. I cried, I yelled, I jumped up and down but to no avail. Suddenly a voice said, "May I help you ma'am?" My mom said yes, and afterwards she grabbed me, with the help of my aunt and the barber. They secured me in the chair of a total stranger that I felt like was about to hurt me. I imagined him squeezing my head until I couldn't cry anymore.

Nothing felt right about the situation. The funny tissue he put around my neck was weird. It seemed as though the cape was buttoned to tight, and the chair was way too big for a kid to be sitting in. As I felt like I was being eaten alive by the oversized chair, this stranger began picking my hair. Every pluck of the pick seemed as though it was with extreme force as the stranger proceeded to pick my hair. I wasn't enjoying this at all, and didn't care who knew it. I remember my mom clamping my arms down so tight I couldn't move them. Finally I gave in. What is a kid suppose to do when his mom, and his aunt are on the stranger's side. I didn't understand it, and I sure didn't like it, but I guess it was right in their eyes. My mom was calling me a good little boy, but I was acting out the complete opposite. I will never forget that day because it seemed as if it was an eternity. "Ok little man, I'm done," the stranger said. It seemed as though the angels began to sing as the barber began to take the cape off and put me into the arms of my mom. My only thought was"I will never be back here again!"

Well I was wrong. It seemed as though my mom took me to that dreadful place much more than I wanted to be there. Years passed by, and I begin to realize my mom was not trying to hurt me. She was only trying to help me. I didn't understand how she would allow a complete stranger to pick and comb through my hair and make me cry in front of everyone.

As I approached my teen years, and the girls began to pay a little more attention to me, the place that was my biggest enemy became my biggest friend. Man, welcome to the Barbershop! I never thought I would be so excited to hop in the chair that I screamed my way out of when I was a kid!

I must admit, a trip to the barbershop became a journey into conversation, and information. You didn't have to watch the news, or buy a daily journal. All you had to do was take a trip to the barbershop. Information fresh off the press was spread through the shop daily, at the entrance of each new customer. Really, new customer, new news! The barbershop is one of a few places you can go and always learn something new. It didn't matter if you were a republican, or democrat, believer, or atheist, black, or white, inner city, or suburb citizen. There was some sort of news for everyone. All it would cost you was a listening ear. Some chatter was enjoyable to hear and always gave you a good laugh. Chatter such as, political debates, sports news and bets. The newest jokes, cracks, and who can forget all the lies that found a feeble pair of ears to occupy.

Men came in from all walks of life. In the shop you could find teachers, plumbers, electricians, coaches, doctors, lawyers, gangbangers, pastors, as well as city leaders. They all gathered together in one room, for one thing, and that was a haircut! I find that amazing to see the man with the most money had to sit in the same seat as the man that made the least money. The pastor had to sit in the same seat as the troubled gangster. The democrat had to sit in the same seat as the republican, and the police officer had to take comfort in the same chair as the ex-criminal. The barbershop was a place that could bring leverage like that to all, and make all feel equal! Thug talk, pastoral counseling, political talk, macho talk, it didn't' matter, it was all mixed into the atmosphere at the same time. Sometimes it could get really heated though with all the debating and joking, to the point you could just about countdown until fight time! Somebody ego was crushed, or someone else's manhood was challenged.

Whatever the situation would be, some conversations were dead end roads. Once you go down them, you couldn't get out no matter how hard you tried! Other conversations were not too inviting, such as overhearing someone's bedroom business, curse words that I didn't know existed, and how can I forget the dirt wrenched names women were given on a daily basis. Once these conversations were brought up, everyone looked at you to co-sign as though they were right. Oh man, don't even bring up religion. You haven't seen a religious war until you experience one in the barbershop. Most of the time it would be people that didn't know the first thing about spiritual principles, but they were found leading the debate. I thought religious wars were bad in the church, but they can't touch a religious debate in the barbershop. Trust me; they can get real nasty in the shop. Real nasty! They say the biggest hypocrites are found in the church. Well I like to beg to differ! The barbershop houses the best hypocrites by far! There is no hypocrite, like one found in the barbershop. It doesn't matter if they are the barber, or the customer. There are some pretending, wanna-be people on this earth! Testosterone is bouncing off the walls at speeds you can only imagine, and no one will never except that their point of view is wrong! No one is wrong, especially if there are any females amongst the discussion. Men really don't like to be wrong when they are in the company of women.

Things you would assume, that should be taught to you for the first time at home or in a college classroom and you will learn it for the first time in the barbershop. Huh, everything was taught in the barbershop! Street slang, as well as pickup lines was taught. The newest fashion, even to how to cheat on your taxes was also a free class in the shop. You learn how to cook, how to lie, how to cheat, and how to be unfaithful to your family. Did I mention you learn how to steal, how to get a rumor started, all the way down to how to stay out of the doghouse (wife trouble)? So many different perspectives on how to be a man, and what a man should be that it could confuse the average kid. This group is saying a real man can't be with just one woman. Another group is saying, "One woman is all a real man need." Real mean don't cry, real men should cry. Real men don't apologize, and others felt like you had to be a real man if you could apologize. If you looked in close enough, you could see the pain that many men carried, but wore a mask and covered their hurt. Loneliness and frustrations were also covered with a bunch of macho sex talk, or how much they pressed in the gym last weekend.

It was funny to see that some guys hung out at the barbershop all day long just to escape the presence of a nagging wife. Some came in just to be amongst the chatter, and get caught up on the latest news. It is said that women gossip, and true is this saying, but I want to know the masculine terminology for the word gossip. Men gossip just as much as women in the barbershop, we just label it as "kicking it." I often wondered if every husband's wife could know the true conversations their husband's really indulged in on a daily basis, would they have a home to come to. The man at home and the man at the shop are two different cats! Believe that!

I perceive some shops like a prison yard. Prisoners gather on the yard to compare muscles and tats, as well as tell lies about unborn fantasies. Once someone is crossed the wrong way, in comes the instigators and out comes the shanks. Same thing in the shop, the only difference is you are free to leave whenever you wish.

I began cutting hair when I was 24 years of age. I was a bit forced into learning how to cut hair when I was forced to cut my own hair. My cousin was my barber for years but when I moved from Wilmington I didn't allow anyone else to cut my hair. With this being the case, my hair grew and grew. I remember having to go to church one night and I was refusing to go without a haircut. I drove to buy a pair of clippers and decided to cut my own hair. I must say it didn't look like my cousin's cut however I did make it to church that night. I received a couple of compliments and the rest is history. I began cutting a few family members as well as a few friends from time to time. My task in the beginning wasn't too stressful. I ran across a couple of minor situations but not anything that caused any stress. Time passed by and I became a licensed barber at the age of 33, and boy did the stress increase! Everything that was already discussed, I now witnessed it on a day-to-day basis! Once you get behind that barber's chair as a career, it's a lot different than sitting in the chair every week or two to get a haircut. You get to see the entire field, and watch every play as they unfold. You find out that you soon become a friend, a counselor, a leader, a mediator and much more to many customers.

Over the years of cutting hair, I began to notice a pattern of habitual things that was practiced by most customers every day. Some of these habits are funny, some are pitiful and some are unbelievable. I decided to put together this book of 101 things your barber/stylist hates but may never tell you, and pray that as every barber read, he/she will find a window in your busy schedule to laugh and develop a sense to know you are not out there alone. On the contrary, my aim is that as the customer will read this book, they will see themselves and began to correct some of this oblivious behavior, or do something about what they may already be aware of. Sit back, relax, and as you began to read, if you come across something that you feel like it would bring a smile on one of your fellow barbers/stylists face, please don't hesitate to share this book with them so they could find an extra laugh throughout their busy day as well. I would like to thank you for your purchase, and your time you have allowed me to share with you. In all the places throughout the world, there is no place like the barbershop!

A merry heart maketh a cheerful countenance: but by sorrow of the heart the spirit is broken.

-Proverbs15:13(KJV)

A merry heart does good like a medicine: but a broken spirit dries the bones.

-Proverbs 17:22(KJV)

I'm grateful and overjoyed that God granted me with the prowess to birth this writing. The primary intent of this writing was to help lead you into laughter that will be responsible for healing the very place(s) you are hurt and broken in. I pray that you will not find offence in any of the content written herein. It was never meant to cause any hurt but only healing through the medicine of laughter. So sit back and relax while you live, love and laugh!

ONE

The Oblivious Parent

If you know your child is a trip at home, you know they are going to be a trip in the public. I don't understand, and may never understand, why a mother/father will bring their untrained, unthankful, and disrespectful kids into the barbershop and act all oblivious about their behavior. You know everywhere you take him he cuts up. In Wal-Mart the kid is eating grapes that you know you are not going to pay for. He uses the bathroom wherever he wants to and you think it's funny. He comes out the china buffet with the people silver ware, out of school with a pocket full of toys, out of the doctor's office with the stethoscope. Must I go on? Your child cuts up, and you know it. You allow him to act unseemly at home, and then expect him not to embarrass you in public. PLEASE!!! There's no need of you acting like you don't know why Lil Johnny Polka Dot is always running around hitting everybody. You think it's cute

1

when he is yelling out cuss words at his barber and everyone else he comes in contact with. He is only acting out what he sees and carrying out the behavior you never correct at home. That's' all right though, if you don't want to correct him, I got something for Lil Polka Dot. There is more than one way to skin a cat. A Wahoo McDaniel or Black Jack Mulligan claw or even a tap on the bottom of the neck with a pair of warm clippers will straighten him out.

Parents, please stop acting oblivious to your misbehaved children. The barber is more upset at your oblivious behavior than he/she is at your child cutting up. Wake up! Everybody can't be lying. You've called your daycare a lie, your church a lie, and your job and family a lie. You have even fallen out with good friends over them telling you about Lil Polka Dot's behavior. Your child cuts up and you know it! I speak for myself, and for every barber/stylist out there. Straighten this out at home, and you will see a major difference in the public. Peace out!

TWO

The Silent Parent

Are you kidding me? You mean to tell me, you are just going to sit there and watch your child give me a hard time and not say or do anything about it. I remember cutting a little guy's hair a couple of years ago. He was about 7, or 8 years old, and believe it or not, this was his first haircut. His mom said she never cut it and decided to grow out dread locks. His locks grew very strong and they had much length as well. Out of the blue she got tired of them and was ready to have them cut. Mind you, this was a Saturday and I was preparing to go home when they walked into the shop. I saw the locks but I thought he was going to get a quick line and be gone. I knew I could line him up in less than 2-3 minutes and be out of there. Legs throbbing, back and knees hurting, I agreed to give him a line so I thought.

All the other barbers began to laugh and crack

jokes, when they heard me get the shock of my life! The mother said, "We are cutting his locks off today". I replied, "Can you say that again". Oh boy, you should have heard the barbershop explode with laughter. Sure enough, she said it again, "We are cutting his locks off today." Tired and all, I began to unpack my clippers and have the little boy sit down. I had to cut the locks with my shears, untangle what was under the locks, shampoo and condition his head, dry his head, and then comb through it. Are you tired yet, because I was exhausted, and I get tired all over again just thinking about it? How about when I was shampooing his hair, the little guy started screaming and trying to kick me. As a matter of fact, one or two of his kicks got me pretty good.

Remember now, this is not a two year old. This boy was about 8 and his kicks came with force. I wanted to scream while I was washing his hair but I held myself together. He kicked, he screamed, he swung, he cursed, he called me names, and how about the mother said absolutely nothing! Can you please say something is what was running through my head, but she never did. I don't know if parents are burned out, or just don't care, but please don't allow your child to go into the barber shop and rip it into pieces and you just turn away as if nothing is happening. The silent parent makes me wonder who is really running things. Say something please!

THREE

The Resister

Whenever you find out why people come to get a haircut, and a clipper shave, but resist the very thing you are trying to do, please call me at 777-9311, Lol! Speaking from a barber's perspective, if you are a customer, and your barber is trying to tilt your head back to cut the hairs from under your neck, please don't resist.

I believe every barber have, or had a customer who had a stiff neck, and didn't give you any play, or slack when you tried to push his chin back to get the shave finished. It's like they feel like if they tilt back, they will pass out or something. Lol! I don't know if the bone in their neck can't move, or if they just want to be in control, or better yet just stubborn. Why did you come to the shop if you don't want to cooperate?

In the shop we use to always shout out "we got a resister", and then another barber will say "quit resisting man, quit resisting!" It was hilarious. Every barber would fall out laughing but the customer would be in the dark to what's so funny. Sir, can I have your attention. If you go to the barbershop, that is saying you trust someone else to take care of your grooming. The only question I have is "why do you go to resist what your barber is trying to do?" Stop resisting and things will run a lot smoother for you, and for your barber!

FOUR

The Mirror Watcher

Attention all barbers/cosmetologists, on a scale of one to ten, ten being the greatest, how much would you say you dislike someone to sit in your chair, and watch the mirror to see your every move? My guess is 11. Although it's not on the scale, 11 is my answer. First of all, I've been cutting your hair for how many years? Second of all, it's hard to mess up a baldhead. And third of all, you're not that cute!

I have at least two or three customers, which I have been cutting for years that just like to hold onto the mirror and look in it after every stroke of the clipper. Come on man, if I haven't messed you up after all these years, what makes you think I will this time. What customers don't understand is, the barber/cosmetologist signature is upon their head, and we don't want our name bad so we have to give you a nice cut each time. No lie, I have a customer that gets a bald head, and he looks in the mirror the entire time he is getting it cut like he is examining my skills or something. Sometimes I have to laugh at myself because I turn the chair at an angle where he can't see anything but the wall; Lol. I can feel his anticipation and restlessness to be turned back around but I ignore it. I don't know when, but one day the mirror watcher will be delivered from his fears, and his perspective of himself being beautiful. Lol!

FIVE

The Talker

Is it possible for you to be quiet for a minute? As s/he is waiting, when s/he sits in the chair, and when s/he is finished, all s/he does is talk. Most of the time s/he is in the dark and has no clue to what s/he is talking about his or herself! There is no way in the world you can always have that much to say. Just to give you the heads up as a customer, if you want your beard or flat iron to be on point, and your mustache not to be cut off, or your goatee to be tight, stop talking for a minute or two. Nobody doesn't want to hear all that craziness you're talking about anyway. Spare me the headaches please. I never thought I would run across a man who just keeps going, and going, and going until I started cutting hair. I can somewhat understand women but it is absolutely amazing to run across men that talk more. It's almost like they know they talk too much, but they can't help it. They try to stop, bless their heart, but its way too much going on in their head and they just have to go where their head is taking them.

I can recall one time I was lining a customer's mustache, and I asked him if he could stop talking for a minute. He said ok, but his lip was trembling, and it was killing him that he had to be quiet. He finally couldn't handle it, and had to say something. I almost ripped his mustache off, and go figure, he was wondering why. If you are a customer reading this book, its ok to talk, you just got to know when to chill out!

SIX

The Green Hand

I remember when I was a kid watching cartoons such as Scooby Doo, and Tom and Jerry. Every so often something use to smell really bad on the show, and a green stream of smoke would begin to arise until it took the shape of a hand. This hand would then travel under the nose of the different characters bringing them to their knees because of the smell. Ladies and gentlemen, the green hand still lives, and cartoon has made it a reality. Coming out from the pit of the stomach marches the thumb, the pinky, and then the rest of the crew that makes up "the green hand". I'm surprised some customers are not charged when they talk because they have murdered many hairs in their barber/stylist nose, and have caused others to literally throw up. Literally!!

I remember a barber I worked with use to tell me about a customer he had with bad breath. I never believed him until one day I was cutting hair, and got a whiff to go across my nose. I literally started choking and coughing. The funny part was the customer with the green hand was getting his hair cut in the chair next to me, but the barber spent him around when he started talking to let me smell the breeze. Boy oh boy did I ever smell it. It was like a horror, or sci-fi film where everything slowed down and all you heard was music, as you were under attack.

We all use to joke on creating a team called the spitfires. We had the starting lineup, the bench, even down to the coaches, and all the boys spit serious fire when they talk. One was so bad, every time he came into the shop he went straight to the candy dish but it never helped. We all laughed that the peppermint melted as he was in motion of putting it into his mouth. If you know your breath stink, don't talk in the barber chair, just smile and nod. I couldn't help but think, does your wife ever tell you about your breath!

SEVEN

The Non-Tipper

Some people want everything for nothing! To be as picky as some customers are, you would think after they pick you to death about every little detail, that they would tip you real good. Not so! It almost reminds me of Chris Rock in I'm Gonna Get You Sucker. A movie back in the late 80's. He worried the man, asked the man a million questions, and misled the man to think he had a decent paying customer. After all of the worrying, he asked to order one rib, not a full order, just one rib, and asked if the soda could be poured in his hand for a dime. After all the begging, he pulled out a knot of money, and asked "you got change for a hundred?" I can name several customers exactly like that, but I will spare them the embarrassment.

After years of cutting them on a weekly basis, hearing their complaints, listening to their lies, counseling them with their problems, smelling their bad breath, and fighting through their greasy hair, the least they could do is give you a couple of extra dollars every now and then. Instead, they give you a twenty and stand there without blinking, until all their change is collected. In most cases, I haven't faced this problem with many female customers. Most of the time it's the stingy husband or male figure! Lol. Or some single man who just refuses to give you a dime extra after you have slaved over his head and made him look halfway decent for his Kmart family pictures. It was the haircut you gave him that got him the job, your haircut that got him the date, and your haircut that gave him his swag back, but still and all he refuse to say thank you with a tip. Come on man!

EIGHT

The Confused/Surprised one about their Dandruff

I f your barber have cut your hair a thousand times, and each time your dandruff fell from your head like snow, why do you act surprised about this each time. I promise you, I have a customer who act so surprised when dandruff fills his lap every time I brush his hair. It makes me laugh inside when he began to shake the cape and say things like "Is your brush clean?," or "Is that falling out of my hair?" Yeah right! They are so shame to the fact that their hair stays dirty, that they will go all out to try to put the blame on you as though you don't keep your combs and brushes clean.

Listen ma'am or sir, all it takes is two to three minutes to wash your hair before coming to the shop. Stop acting surprised when snow began to fall out your head. If you want to save yourself some shame, and some acting, the next time you even think you are going to the barbershop, please get the snow out.

NINE

The Shorter

You remember back in the day when your uncle use to ball up a few ones and put them in your hand and act like he gave you a lot of money. This is how some customers are. They knew they were a few dollars short before they sat down in your chair. As you take your time cutting their hair, they are probably cracking up inside because they know they are about to do you real dirty! I can only imagine the thoughts that bum rush through their head during each stroke of the clipper.

The haircut is done and the barber now moves on to the edge up. About this time the customer have had ample time to tell his barber he is a few dollars short today. Nope, he yet closes his eyes and enjoys the sound of the trimmers tightening up the last piece of his line. "Alright my man" says the barber after dusting him off, wiping him with astringent, and spraying good smelling oil sheen in his hair. He jumps out the chair in confidence. "Cool" he replies, and then grab your hand, shake it, and put about nine ones in your hand and head out the door like he is rushing to an appointment or something. At the time it feels like it's well more than enough to cover his service, but when you count it, you realize he got you again. Your next customer is already in the chair, and the one that beat you is driving off. Some people are not going to do right no matter what. When he comes back and you refuse him service, he will say you are doing him wrong. Reality check, if you can't do it in Burger King, or McDonald's, don't do it to your barber or stylist! Pay up or tell us in advance that you are short.

TEN

The "Can I Get You Next Week" Customer

Yes some barbers are blessed to make a good comfortable living, but just because you see them with a knot of money doesn't give you the right to feel like they don't need your twenty dollars. Sometimes people think a person that has a lot is not in need of anything else. I believe some millionaires and billionaires are often hurt. Reason is because they are frequently overlooked during holidays and birthdays. Most people think they are ok so why give them a gift.

Every other Friday, me and a couple of other barbers use to prepare ourselves for the best laugh of the day as we spotted the dreadful customer storming across the parking lot, trying to rush in to get a last minute haircut that he knew he wasn't going to pay for until the following week. We use to make fun of his barber because he knew he was getting ready to get beat! Sure enough, he would get a nice cut and a sharp line as always. He is ready for the weekend and has already made plans. At the last moment he would always say "Can I take care of you next week?" We would all fall-out laughing and our weekend was made with that laugh.

It would be a good idea to ask before you take the seat next time. That could have very well been the funds we were in need of to pay an important bill. Just because you see your barber/stylist with a lot doesn't necessarily mean they have a lot.

ELEVEN

The Important One

It's a fact that all men are created equal, but often times others seem to miss this simple concept. If you want to see some Miami Vice action in real life, spend a couple of hours at the barbershop. Especially on the weekend. If you can use your imagination, you would literally hear the intro music, and see doves flying out from some customer's cars and following behind them as they approach the shop in slow motion.

I wanted to hire a couple of bodyguards for several customers that I saw stepping across the parking lot with their palm pilot, books and highlighters as if they read every hour on the hour. Really man! Are you really that important that you need three cell phones, and have to pull them out in front of everyone and make sure they see them all. Nobody's calling you that much. Last I heard, President Obama only had one phone and really didn't like talking on that one. Give it a break and let importance take its course. You don't have to force it.

There is a difference in being important, and wanting to be important. In most cases, people that are important don't want to be. On the contrary, people that want to be important are usually not. Sorry that it works that way bro. Uncross your legs, throw the bookmarkers away, take the doves back to the petting zoo, and be you! Don't settle for being a cheap copy; strive to be that priceless original. No one can beat you, at being you!

TWELVE

The Man that's Always in a Hurry!

One thing I will never understand as a barber is how some customers manage their time. The true currency of life is not money, but time. Wherever we spend the most of our time is the place we spend most of our life. I think customers should be more considerate about coming to the shop always in a hurry. A man that's always in a hurry is a dangerous man, not a busy man. He is dangerous because it shows that he always overbooks his own schedule, and never has time (life) for himself.

My mind takes me back to a customer we all called Cuz. He earned this name faithfully because that's the only thing he called everybody he talked to. As soon as he walked in the shop, someone will say "What's up, Cuz!" he would reply with a big grin on his face, "*Everythang* good, Cuz." Everybody was either cuz, or big daddy. He would also say "You know what I'm saying Big daddy?" The majority of everybody was cuz though. I never saw the day when Cuz was able to come to the shop and just chill and be patient.

He would walk in and before he sat down would say "I'm in a hurry cuz, who can get me?" every so often he would get lucky and a barber would be available to get to him. Many times it didn't work that way. No barber would be available for at least thirty minutes to an hour and sometimes longer than that. We would all watch to see if cuz was going to stay or leave. We saw how much of a hurry cuz was not in because he would sit down and wait like everyone else. Slow down Cuz, and manage your time!

THIRTEEN

The Stalker

t's certainly true that some people elevator doesn't go to the top floor. You have to be really desperate or just plain crazy to do what some customers do to their barbers/stylist. I never thought I would be stalked by anyone until I became a barber. I witnessed with my own eyes, the stalking habits some customers have. It is downright amazing, but disturbing at the same time. I remember being in the bathroom one day at the shop, and all of a sudden there was a knock on the door. I thought some of the fellows were playing around trying to scare me because that's what we use to do at times. I ignored the knock, but they wouldn't let up. I hung in the bathroom a little longer than usual because I thought the boys were trying to scare me when I came out. Finally everything got really quiet so I came out. All the barbers started laughing because staring right in my face was my barbershop stalker. I said, "Come on, man, you got to follow me to the bathroom!"

I believe if the door was unlocked, he would have just opened the door and came in. If you are a customer reading this, please stop stalking your barber. Quit riding through the parking lot real slow like you on "Boyz in the Hood" looking for your barber's car or truck. Quit watching your barber/stylist while they eat lunch, trying to see how many more bites they have left. Just chill out and give the man/woman some space, they will get with you when they can. Stalking is not going to make you get a haircut any faster.

FOURTEEN

The Moon

If you feel a cool breeze on your backside while you are getting a haircut, chances are that your barber is about to get the surprise of his/her life. I don't understand why customers don't feel the urge to cover their body and save everyone else the exposure. I'm sure most barbers have at least one customer who can never find a pair of pants that properly fit. Things you would rather not see are always exposed whenever you take the cape off, to release them out from the chair. Let me tell you my friend, your barber doesn't want to continue to be surprised week after week. If we wanted to see the moon, we know where to look. I have heard the terminology "Eye Candy" but this defeats, and is totally contrary to the meaning of this word.

FIFTEEN

The Last Minute Man

I always thought it was funny to go into a restaurant right before closing time and see the look on the worker's faces while I was placing my order. My respect changed when the shoes were placed on my feet. I don't care how many times you tell certain customers, they will always show up five minutes until closing time.

In many cases, it's the same customer that always acts like you never told him what time you close. He act all surprised when he show up at 2:55 on a Saturday, and you already told him/her several times that you are closing at three. "Three?" "I thought you close at six." I keep telling you we close at six, Tuesday through Friday. You've been coming to this shop for 5 years and still acting like you're confused with the business hours.

After you have cut 25 to 30 heads or more, your legs are burning, your back is tight, your knees are aching, and you had to skip lunch so you wouldn't get too far behind, in comes the last minute customer. Your eyes are on the door and your mind and heart is already home. They come through begging for your services, and out of the kindness of your heart, you cut or style their hair. The funny part is after all that, they refuse to tip. If you are going to continue to be a last minute man, please be considerate and take care of your barber/stylist like they always take care of you.

SIXTEEN

The Taco Meat Man

I understand the realities of life, and that one of those realities is that we will all face times in life when we will have to be in a big hurry. The only thing I'm struggling to understand is why in those times we snatch up anything to put on and make our way to the barbershop. I've witnessed customers with their stomach hanging out the bottom of their shirt, meat bulging out from the side of the "wife beater", hair waving at you out the armpits. Man, put some clothes on please! You wouldn't walk into another place of business like you're at the beach or something.

Around the shop we label this customer as the taco man. We all know what a taco looks like right? It's just a shell with a bunch of meat that's exposed everywhere in it. Meat that's flabby and falling all over the place. No form, no structure, no cares, just meat that's there. I don't know if they feel like they are the smoothest thing going but it sure seems that way. The next time you are in a hurry Mr. /Mrs. /Ms. Customer, grab something other than your little brother or little sister's tee, especially if you are headed to the barber shop. There are enough restaurants that we can go to buy our tacos. We didn't ask for our eyes to abruptly go into shock. If we want taco meat, we know where to go find it!

SEVENTEEN

The Picky One

What is it that fulfills you? Gossip? Peace? Negativity? Unity? Everyone have their personal taste of fulfillment, even if making their barber's life miserable by being overly picky that fulfills them. Some customers point out the smallest things that you almost need to be standing right in their face, or look through a microscope to see. It's like their day will not be complete unless they mess someone else's day up. Some days, there are times when other barbers are complimenting the haircut you just gave a customer, but the customer steady points out your mistakes that are hidden to everyone else but him. It's like he has mistake radar in his head or something.

There was one particular customer that came in the barbershop and was refused service by everyone. It was my first couple of weeks in the shop and I didn't understand it so I offered my help. I was wondering why all the other barbers were grinning and pointing. Boy, did I find out! I didn't find out until the next day, but I sure found out! How about this customer came back in the next week and said I didn't cut their hair correctly. I said, "Ok, let's fix it, sit down." I cut it again, showed the customer the mirror and she agreed it was right.

After the customer left the shop, everyone was laughing. I asked them why they were laughing. They told me, "She does that to everyone; no one can cut her hair right." They said, all of us in here have cut her hair, and it's the same excuse. She just likes to be hard and picky. Weeks went by and she came back in the shop. Most of the barbers were lying about how many they had before her because they knew she wouldn't want to wait. Everybody else ignored her and she walked out mad! Be careful how picky you are, it may come back to haunt you. I would be surprised if she can get a haircut anywhere now because her name is known throughout the city. It doesn't pay to be extra picky!

EIGHTEEN

The Man in Denial

"Ok, this is what I want." "I want it even, but I want to keep it dark, and I want to keep my sideburns long." The barber stares and has to say within, "You're kidding, right?" They carefully explains to the customer how the haircut is already light, how can you keep it dark. "Also, there is no hair in the top, or in the corners." "The only way this is going to be an even haircut is for me to use a straight razor." Here goes the moment of denial. "What are you talking about? I'm not going bald!" I can't understand how a grown man can be in such denial about something as small as losing his hair.

I mean, it's unbelievable to hear, and see some of the denial stories in the barbershop. Some customers walk in with hair around the side and very little hair on the top. We use to joke around in the shop and say, "its one string that's holding it all together." If you hit that one string wrong, everything is going to unravel. I mean, for some customers, their hair is so thin in the top, you can see their scalp smiling and waving at you.

One customer constantly reminds me of when he had a flat top hair cut, and how his hairline always stayed sharp. I believe his mind is still stuck on those years because now he is going bald and still want a sharp hairline. He constantly looks in the mirror when I'm edging him up, to see if it's sharp! I've told him for the past two years, "The darker the hair, the sharper the line." For some reason, he can't comprehend this. To all customers, that will read this book, if you are losing it, man let it go!

NINETEEN

The Man that's Kissing the Sky

I don't support any kind of substance abuse, so please don't take me the wrong way for what I am about to say. If you are going to get high, please do it hours before you come to the barbershop. Some customers seem like they wake up, get blunted up, and head straight to the shop to get a cut. I stopped smoking years ago, but there are times when it felt like I got a buzz from the customer I was cutting. Him, and all his boys that are rolling with him, come in, and change the aroma of the entire shop.

There was one customer in particular that always came in high as a kite. He was always kissing the sky. I use to have to hold my breath at times and even put cologne on my top lip to try to keep the smell under control. On a few occasions, he was so high during the haircut, he had to jump out the chair with the cape on and run next door to the restaurant to get something to drink before he passed out. On one occasion, I must admit, he scared me really good. During the haircut, he dropped his head and was completely silent. He started sweating uncontrollably. He was seconds from passing out. I unbuttoned the cape, took the neck strip off, and he took off running to the bathroom. Everybody in the shop was telling him, "Man, you gonna have to do better than what you're doing."

Unless your barber love to get high himself, it's not cool to flop down in his chair when you are smelling like a pound of weed, giving everybody in the shop a headache. If you are going to do you, please do it hours before you arrive for your haircut. To make things even sweeter, take a shower, brush your teeth, use some mouthwash, and top that off with a piece of gum, or a breath mint. Thank you for doing your barber a favor!

TWENTY

The Text Man

One of the greatest shortcuts in life has also become one of the greatest distractions in life. What is this shortcut you may be asking? This shortcut is called texting. Texting has changed the world in a lot of positive ways. To the person that doesn't like to talk much, he or she may now text. For a quick reminder of an appointment, you can now text. Even for a supermarket list reminder, texting has become a friend of mine. I must admit, technology is making life simple.

On the contrary, there are a lot of negatives attached with the advancing of technology. Texting is responsible for car accidents, stolen attention with a spouse while watching a movie or while trying to enjoy dinner, and is also the leading cause for kids being suspended from school. People are now distracted and preoccupied in church because of texting.

Sad to say, when a customer is texting while he is getting a haircut, it can get very annoying to the barber. Most of the time when you are texting, your head is down because you are looking at your phone. Did you come to get a haircut, or did you come to text that woman or man that is probably seeing someone else anyway. Sometimes it seems as though customers wait until they get in your chair to start texting. I don't know if they feel like it makes the haircut process flow smoother, or if they just like making their barber frustrated by holding their head down. Whatever the case may be, try your best not to text while you are in your barber's chair. If you just have to, learn how to hold the phone up, so your head want have to be hanging down.

TWENTY-ONE

The Phone Talker

There's nothing more annoying than cutting someone's hair that is constantly on the phone. There are some customers that are brilliant enough to switch the phone from ear to ear depending on which side the barber is working on. The funny thing is there are some customers who have no clue that it's time to switch the phone to the other ear. There are some instances when I had to throw the hint by cutting the clippers off and stopping the haircut. Other times I had to just ask him to switch ears.

Sometimes they are on the speaker, sometimes Bluetooth, but most of the time, the phone itself is against their ear. I know barbers are blamed of talking a lot, but in most cases, customers are not considerate to the next man that is waiting. As long as they are in the chair, they don't care how long it takes for their hair to get cut. While they are waiting, you can see the impatience on their face, but they don't have that same mind when it's their turn and they are sitting in the barber's chair. They talk, they laugh, they joke, and they don't care!

If you are a customer and you are reading this book, you must consider how you felt when someone was in the chair talking on the phone slowing down your turn for a haircut. While you are waiting, you are mad, frustrated, and in a hurry. What makes you think its right when you do it to the next man waiting? Don't get me wrong, I'm not saying you have to sit in the barber chair and be silent, but I am saying be considerate, especially when the next man is waiting.

TWENTY-TWO

The 24-Hour, 365 Swag

I didn't think I would ever meet a person that never takes a break from being cool. Cool when they walk, cool when they talk, cool when they drive, they are even cool when they eat! WAY TOO MUCH SWAG! 24 hours a day, 365 days a year. I remember we use to jokingly ask a few customers when they walked in the shop if they ever took a break from being cool. If you really think about it, being cool takes a lot of effort. You have to constantly remember to walk a certain way, lean a certain way, and talk a certain way. Trying to act cool is too much brainwork for me.

There was one young man in my chair that was so cool he didn't want to cough. He kept holding it in and holding it in until he almost choked. He was sitting with his hand over his mouth, and was refusing to allow his cough to interfere with his swag. He was so cool I thought I was going to have to call 911 to report hypothermia. I started laughing inside and shaking my head because it's not that serious man! Please give coolness a break sometimes. You're working cool so much, that "cool" is tired!

I have a few customers that are so cool, one in particular that he can't even sit up straight in the chair while he is getting a haircut. I have to laugh when he sits down and lean to the side in my chair like he is driving down the strip in Myrtle Beach or somewhere. The sad part about it is that all of them are well over 40. Give it up man and let the young boys have it. You might get a better haircut if you can sit up straight in the chair the next time. The minute you get out of your twenties, give cool a break!

TWENTY-THREE

The Grease Head!

Have you ever saw anyone who constantly put grease in their hair on top of grease that was already in their hair and never washed it out. I have another true story for you. I had a customer who was desperately trying to get waves in his hair, that he constantly stacked grease in his hair. Not only did he stack grease in it, but he never washed the old grease out. His hair literally looked silver because of all the dirt and old grease that was in his hair. He was just another joke around the shop. Every time we saw him walking up, someone will say, "Here comes silver".

Man, you're talking about a bittersweet moment. It was sweet because it was a chance to make a little more pocket change. Bitter because I knew it was about to be another tug of war through the grease jungle. One of the biggest barber pet peeve is the guy who has a bunch of grease in his head, and wants a nice even haircut with a tight line. The best way to get a clean even cut with a tight line is to have a clean scalp. Believe me, your barber hates cutting hair that has grease in it. It makes the hair clump together and clogs the clippers up, and also get all the guards stained and filled with grease. If you care anything about your barber, and the way your haircut turns out, wash the grease out and everything will run much smoother. It will also take half the time to cut it and everyone else will be happy for that!

TWENTY-FOUR

The Du-rag Man

The du-rag man flows from the same vein as the one with too much grease in their hair. Reason being is, usually someone who is trying to get waves is more than likely to wear a du-rag. Wearing a du-rag is not the real issue, but the timing in which you take it off is what your barber hates. I'm still trying to figure out why some du-rag customers wait until they are sitting in your chair to start taking it off. Now, not only is your hair full of grease, it's now pressed together because of the du-rag. Customers, please listen to me. If you know you are on your way to the barbershop, don't even put it on. Bring it with you, leave it in the car, and put it on after you get your haircut.

Some customers will sacrifice going bald to keep up with the latest style. I say this because I had a couple of customers that didn't understand why their hair was falling out in a perfect curve in the back of their head. I already knew why, but I still asked, "How often do you wear your du-rag?" Of course their response was "all the time." I tried to explain to them, that the string that is used to tie the rag on your head is too tight, and it's suffocating your hair follicles. Your hair can't breathe, and that's why it's falling out. They just replied "Oh," and put the du-rag on directly after the cut. Risking going bald for a style. You got to be kidding me man!

TWENTY-FIVE

The Man That Think He Knows Your Next Move

I'm sure most barbers go through this with one or more of their customers. While you are cutting a customer's hair, they are already tilting their head, or raising their head, or already moving their face in the direction they think you are about to go. I'm not even thinking about trimming your mustache and you are already folding your lips together expecting me to do it. I don't know about most barbers, but for me, there is no routine pattern I follow on every head I cut. Some customers must think so because they can get ahead of you and assume that they know your next move. Um, excuse me, who have the clippers, you or me? Thank you for wanting to assist your barber, but please allow him/her to promote each move of the haircut or facial trim. There have been customers that almost got done real dirty because they felt like they knew the next move of their barber. What I mean by this is, they almost got a gap, or got something cut slam off because of their sudden move due to prejudgment of their barber's next move. If you are a customer, and you are reading this book, chill out, relax, and take advantage of being groomed. If your barber needs you to move, believe me, he/she will let you know.

TWENTY-SIX

The Barber Poster Man

E very time I think about the barber poster man I have to laugh because it's one of the funniest things we joked at one another about. I had a customer that walked me to the poster that many barber shops hung up to show the various types of cuts that were available. I mean every time he came in he would say, "Come, let me show you what I want." While in route to the poster, all the other barbers use to laugh and point because they knew how I felt walking with the same customer every single time to the poster.

While they were laughing it seemed as though everything slowed down, and we were moving in slow motion. It felt like I was walking the green mile. In most cases, this customer would get to the board and almost look at every haircut. He didn't even care how long he was there, or consider whomever else I had waiting. Sometimes he would make up his mind and point at the cut he would like, wait a while and then say, "Ah, no I think I want it like this one, no, like this one." Every time I saw him walking in I would already prepare myself for the walk, the laughing and pointing, and everything else that came along with the barber poster man. Give your barber and yourself a break sometime, and come in without the extras, and the drama. Just explain your haircut and sit down.

TWENTY-SEVEN

The Man That Turns the Chair with His Feet, when it's Not Time

I f the barbershop is crowded, and every barber chair is occupied, there is bound to be at least ten to fifteen different conversations going on at the same time. Sometimes the guy that you are cutting will try to find interest in as many conversations as he can. This can get frustrating to a barber because without warning, the customer uses his feet to turn the chair in the direction of the conversation that best interest him. I can't speak for all barbers, but this is one of my pet peeves. I cannot stand it when my customer turns the chair around by himself, especially when he turns it without giving me a warning. I don't know what runs through the head of customers sometimes, but I can't picture myself sitting in a barber's chair, grip the floor with my feet, and turn the chair where I want it, and when I want to.

Sometimes you are tempted as a barber to

almost give the customer whiplash, and jerk the chair back into its original position. I have caught myself grabbing the chair, and was seconds away from catching a whiplash charge, but checked myself at the last minute and politely moved the chair back into place. I know you may be use to being in charge, but when you are in your barber's chair, you must learn how to lose control, and let your barber be the pilot at the moment. After you are released from the chair, you can have your position of control back. But until then, stop turning my chair!

TWENTY-EIGHT

The Fake Barber

I can't count how many of my customers have told me that they are barbers or they at one time use to cut hair. I don't know if they feel like they will get a better haircut, or if they feel like they are intimidating you when they sit in your chair and say, "I cut hair too." "I use to cut in New York; I use to cut in Philly." I use to, I use to, or I am, please stop it! You don't pick up any brownie points with your barber by saying you are a barber.

I have a customer that always ask me, why I didn't do this first, why I didn't do that last, what made me cut against the grain, and so on. He finally told me he was a barber, but the funny part about it was he didn't know a blade from a guard. I just played along with it, as I believed he was a barber. I knew he couldn't cut hair if he had to in order to save his life. Most of the time when I finished he would say how tight the cut was. I would just respond soberly "appreciate it". Once again, if you are a customer that is reading this book, you don't get any brownie points or any discounts for saying you are a barber. So stop making up stories! Thank you! And by the way, if you're that good, cut your own hair!

TWENTY-NINE

The Lip Licker

May you tell me how many times are you going to lick your lips? If you lick your lips one more time, I'm going to cut my clippers off. I don't know what make a man like his lips so much that he has to lick them every other second. I don't think it ever occurred to me how much some brothers lick their lips until I started cutting hair. I don't know if their lips are really that dry, if it's just a habit, or if they think they are the greatest gift to the shop at the time they are there.

I can vaguely understand if a guy is licking his lips when a lady of his interest is in the room, but when the room is full of men, and you are in the barber's chair, you got to help me understand bro. What's with the lip licking? I mean every other second. You can barely line their mustache up because they can't keep their mouth still.

Sometimes I just want to ask them if they need

a minute with their self, or if they need me to call their wife or girl friend to rescue them. I promise you, I believe they have to drink all kinds of power-up drinks when they leave because they have to be dehydrated after all the water they put on their lips. From the time you start the haircut, until the time you finish, you get a chance to witness a man in love with himself. You must trust me; the sight is not cool at all. Get you some chap stick brotha, or maybe even a lady barber, she may want to watch you lick your lips, but as long as you have a man for a barber, try to keep your tongue in your mouth.

THIRTY

The Cussing Sailor

I don't know where the terminology come from as far as "cussing sailor", but if it's true that sailors love to cuss, every naval academy that's missing sailors need to check the barber shop because there are quite a few in there that know how to cuss real good. I know about the NFL, but I didn't know there was a NCL (National Cussing League).

I remember this one customer in particular. Every time we would see his gold Cadillac pull up, every barber would take off running. Nobody wanted to deal with his nasty mouth. Every other word would have to be a word that you probably couldn't find in the dictionary. Some guys do it because they think they need to in order to be cool or accepted. Others do it just to do it. The sad part is, some do it, and have been doing it so long, they don't even know when they do it. At some point it would get out of control, and we would address it, and he would ask, "What did I say?" He really would be clueless that he just used every letter in the alphabet, but in the wrong way.

THIRTY-ONE

The Deebo

"**W**hat you got on this 40, Craig?" You remember Deebo don't you? Every now and then his personality pops up in the neighborhood barbershop through a customer or two. Reminiscing on one customer in particular that came in the shop every so often. No barber wanted to fool with him because he was always sending out his little threats about hurting whoever mess his cut up. He was a pretty big guy, and chiseled all over. He looked crazy, and always had this lil swag of toughness. I remember shaping his beard up one day. I showed him the mirror, and he said it looked good. I carefully let him out of the chair with a sigh of relief. The next time he came in, about two weeks later, he said he will never let me cut him again because I messed him up. He went to another barber, and I was so glad because I didn't want to cut him again.

That day when he left, all the barbers started laughing. They said he say that about anybody that cut his hair. He just like acting like Deebo because he is chiseled. Another occasion, he came in the shop and allowed one of the barbers to shave his head with a straight razor. Everybody was holding their breath with every stroke of the razor. He nicked him, blood started flowing, and I started praying. He got up and said, "I should kill you fool!" I believe the thing that saved this barber was the fact that he was deaf. Dee-bo just stood up, rubbed his head, and started cussing and walked out. Be careful, because we all know what happen to Deebos. There is always a "Craig" ready to knock him out in the end!

THIRTY-TWO

The Sweater

There is nothing worse than a guy sitting in your chair that can't stop sweating. It's almost like he just got finished running a marathon, and ran straight to the barbershop to sit in your chair. He comes in and sweat is dripping everywhere. The more he wipe, the more he sweats. There was one guy that came to the shop and he would always be sweating. We all made fun of him because no matter if it was hot, or cold outside, he came in sweating.

Only barbers will understand how annoying it can get as you are trying to cut a person's hair that's constantly sweating. Everyone wants a good haircut, and a tight line, but everyone don't understand that some things the customer does makes it hard for their wishes to be accomplished. I know sometimes you as the customer can sometimes get in a hurry, but you have to understand sweat is a barber's enemy. Try cooling down, and getting your sweat under control before flopping down in your barber's chair, he will thank you for it.

Yes something as small as sweat plays a part in the outcome of your haircut. If you want a real tight line, you have to do something about all that sweat. The trimmers are crying as they lay on top of your wet forehead trying to make a sharp line. The hair is being pulled instead of cut, and your barber is getting more and more frustrated by the minute. Bring a cold rag, or an ice pack. Get that sweat under control, and get the best haircut and line you ever got. You as the customer owe me for this tip!

THIRTY-THREE

The Nicotine

Nicotine and I are not good friends. Every time I smell cigarette smoke, I get really dizzy and lightheaded. I really don't even like to see people smoke; especially women. Every now and then I get a customer that makes me feel like I'm smoking, the entire time I'm cutting his hair. The nicotine is so strong as though he just finished eating a pack of cigarettes. The smell seems as though it's coming through his pores as he breath.

When I'm cutting someone's hair like that, I wish I could hold my breath throughout the duration of the haircut but I can't. I've tried eating peppermints, putting cologne on my top lip, and even spraying air freshener. Nicotine is just a hard smell to defeat, but I shouldn't have to try to defeat it while you are sitting in my chair. You, as the customer should try to make your barber as comfortable as you possibly can in order to get the best haircut you deserve.

I know barbers because I happen to be one. I say that because I know the reality of rushing through a haircut because of the smell of nicotine that is too overwhelming.

THIRTY-FOUR

The Two Year Old Fade/Taper

Every time you see a baby come through the door, there is a part of you that automatically cringes. Reason being is, you know your work is cut out for you, you just don't know how badly. You always hope for the best when you see a child and his mother, or father come through the door, but chances are you are in for a struggle. The kid is already looking funny and examining everything that's around him, and now you have to pump yourself up in order to cut his hair. It gets even worse if it's his first haircut. I know of a couple of barbers that hung up their clippers and gave barbering up because their nerves couldn't take the threat of the children.

Cutting a child's hair can be a double edge sword. The only thing is you never know which end of the blade you will get from week to week. One week you cut them, they are laughing, sitting still, and cooperating. The next week you get to see Jason, and Freddy Kruger come out at the same time. One of the biggest challenges is when one of the parents ask, "may you cut him a fade?" Or, "may you taper the sides?" Another one is when they want their two year old that will not sit still to get a line or edge-up. The funny part is they see he will not sit still, and they refuse to help assist you in holding him. I know the fade, the taper, and the line may be cute on your two-year-old, but if you know he refuse to sit still, please show his barber some love and say "Let's wait until he is a little older."

THIRTY-FIVE

The Eyebrow Raiser

I have yet to figure out why some customers like to raise their eyebrows while they are getting a line. I have examined, and watched to see if they do it during the time you are cutting their hair. Nine times out of ten they will not do it. It seems as if they know what they are doing, and just like to wait for the most imperfect time to raise their eyebrows. I have messed up several hairlines in my days of cutting hair because of this eyebrow raising technique that many customers have adapted to. I know I speak for many barbers and myself across the globe that has been victims to the eyebrow raiser. Kids do it, fathers do it, even down to mothers when they are getting their eyebrows arched do it.

Many times if it wasn't for the alertness of the barber to pull the trimmers, or razor back at the right time, there will be a bunch of upset customers. But who will really be the blame, the customer, or the barber? They raise their eyebrows almost as if they were saying, "Huh?" I believe some of them don't even recognize that they are doing this frustrating habit. If this is you, and you know you are doing it, please get a grip on yourself and stop it. If you have no idea that you are doing it, maybe you can ask your barber. Trust me, they will tell you!

THIRTY-SIX

The Liar

We've all told some pretty good lies in our days, but you haven't met a liar like a barbershop liar! There are some customers who go way out, and overboard with the lies they tell. I have heard it all from, "I own a mansion in Burlington N.C." to "Jay Z is my cousin" to "I helped write the script to this movie." There was one guy who came around selling DVDs and cd's on a regular. He came around to try to make an extra dollar, but I had begun to think he came around just to tell a lie. It's as though this was how he got satisfaction and fulfillment out of the day. It seemed as if he didn't tell a lie he wouldn't be happy.

I mean he just came in shooting them off, one after another. Small ones, to medium size ones, all the way down to lies that were so huge, they couldn't fit in the biggest city if they were shrunk down to size. I mean they just didn't make any sense at all. We all use to say, "Come on man, I didn't ask for this!" "It would be different if I asked you to lie to me, than for you to just fire them at me without warning." Just picture someone walking in your shop with a machine gun and started firing as soon as they walked in. A lot of people are going to get hit. That's how it is with the liar; every ear that's listening gets hit.

One day he came in and told us he and a few of his homeboy's went to the super bowl in Atlanta back in 2005. He said they let him in free and he was able to do what he wanted to while he was there at the game. It gets worse, because he told us that he was hanging out with Gabrielle Union and she was all over him. LOL, uncaused for right. You will be amazed at what people will do for attention. Especially in the barbershop. Stop lying, man!

THIRTY-SEVEN

The Bad News Man

I have learned over the years that everybody lights up the room. Some when they come, others when they go. It just so happens that some people don't know which category they fit in. We had so much fun in the shop laughing at this guy we called the "Bad News Man." Every single time he came into the shop, he was telling us some bad news. He would say things like, "I was walking in Wal-Mart you know, and I hurt my leg." or "I was driving my kids to school, and the tire came off the truck." You could never get any good news out of him no matter how hard you tried. We got so use to him and his bad news, whenever he walked in we would say, "What happened bad today?" That's really not a good way to be known as the guy who promotes bad news.

It didn't matter what time of day it was, he would bring the bad news. Sometimes we would tell him that it was too early to hear bad news, and he would still say, "My dog ran away today!" Someone would then say, "You got to get out of here with all this bad news." Some days you could be going through enough bad news in your own personal life and guess who would come in? You guessed it, the bad news man. "Man I was running across the street and my leg fell off." Sad, but it's the sad truth. If you are a bad news individual, and you are reading this book, please stop spreading your bad news like you're spreading mayonnaise on a sandwich. Your barber has enough problems of his/her own.

THIRTY-EIGHT

The Kid That Cleans His Face with the Chair Cloth

If I had the permission to pull off my belt and whip some of the little kids that come through the shop, I will gladly take full advantage of the opportunity. It gives me a very small sense of pleasure when I imagine myself whipping the ill-mannered kids that cut up in the barber's chair.

One of the most disturbing things a kid can do is try to wipe hair off of his face with the chair cloth. I don't know why they do it but it never fail. They get a little hair on their face from the haircut, but then they take the chair cloth and wipe their face trying to get the little bit off, but only put a bunch more on. You can show them the mirror and try to explain to them that they are putting more hair in their face than they are taking off. No matter how you try to explain it, they just don't seem to get it. Sometimes I think they prefer to have a face full of hair so they will have something to complain about. Sometimes I will just let them do what they do, and leave it there.

It can really get on a barbers last nerve to have a child sitting in the chair swarming and constantly trying to get hair off of their face with hair. The sad part about it is that the parent never says anything to stop their child. If you are a parent that's reading this book, please help assist your barber while he/she is cutting your child's hair. It will make it better for them and the child.

THIRTY-NINE

The No Show, No Call

A lot of barbershops are moving into taking appointments from their customers. This could be a good system that will save everyone a lot of time if it is executed properly. The only problem is, it takes commitment from both sides in order to make a plan work.

If a customer makes an appointment with you, and you don't show up as the barber, you will be talked about, called sorry, and may even get fired as being a person's barber. But what happen when you are the customer and you make an appointment and don't show or call, you think nothing of it. I guess no one ever told you, so I'm telling you now, you can't look for commitment from someone and you don't give commitment back. If you feel like it's right for your barber to show up, or at least call you when he can't make it, you should feel like it's right for you to do the same. I speak for all barbers and stylists on this matter. Please do right and call if you know you are not going to make it to your appointment on time or not make it at all. Do unto others as you want them to do unto you.

FORTY

The Second Haircut Man

"Yeah, let me get a one and a half against the grain and round it off in the back." One of the first things I learned in barber school was cut a little bit off, show the customer the mirror, and then continue after they approve or disapprove. I have learned this simple technique will save you a lot of time, and a lot of frustration. There are times I still forget to show the customer the mirror until the end of the haircut. I mean, I give them what they ask for, but after they look in the mirror they ask, "Can we go a little shorter?" You've got to be kidding me. There is nothing else more frustrating to have several customers waiting and someone in your chair that wants a second haircut.

I try to avoid this situation the best I could but every now and then I can forget. It seems as though we should be able to charge them twice because we cut their hair twice. They can care less about how many people are waiting; as long as they are in the chair they are good. Let me ask you Mr. Customer, if you get your haircut twice, should you pay twice? Maybe all barbers need to get together and enforce a new rule and stick to it. If you get a haircut the length that you explained, and after the cut is finished, you look in the mirror and want to go lower, you have to pay for another haircut. This rule will make a lot of customers be more considerate, and it will save barbers and hair stylists much needed time!

FORTY-ONE

The Faithful Explainer

Sometimes I think a lot of people that come to the barbershop are very forgetful. I say this because of how they so easily forget that you have been cutting their hair for years, but every time they get in your chair, they feel like they have to explain what they want. They sit down and say, "This is what I want." After I stand there for a while and act like I'm listening, I say "Ok, just like last time, right?" They always say, "Yeah, like last time." Is that forgetful characteristics or what? You know how a forgetful person always seem to forget he/she just put their keys in their pocket minutes ago but shortly after they are looking all around the house for them. They say there is something that puts everybody in their own class, and I guess this is the dividing factor that comes into play for several customers. I guess some customers get joy from faithfully explaining what kind of haircut they want. I don't want to be the person to rob them from their satisfaction so I have learned to just let them do what they do, and afterwards give them the same haircut that I've been giving them for years!

There was one customer I will never forget. He wore a small semi-box style hair cut. It was something I wanted to see get cut off, but he thought the world of it. You would probably have to fight him if you cut his box off because he really loved it. Every single time he would point at the corners and tell you how he wanted them rounded off, he would tell you not to line him up in the front, and on and on. And we would always respond, "Just like last time, right?" He would say, "Yes, just like last time." He was truly the faithful explainer.

FORTY-TWO

The Lingerer

I know without a doubt, there are a lot of customers that don't have a job. I mean, they can't because of how long they hang around at the shop and just linger after they get a haircut. Don't get me wrong, I have nothing against someone that wants to get involved with barbershop chatter, or be entertained by a joke or two. That's totally okay, it's the guy that wants to linger around your chair and talk, and talk, and talk. After they get a cut, they can see you have someone else waiting. They get up; pay you, and stand there talking. Most of the time they are talking about nothing! You try your best to throw hints, and you keep looking away letting him know you are not interested in what he is saying, or to let him know you are busy. They don't get the hint so they keep lingering, and talking.

I don't want the next customer to feel uncomfortable while they are getting a haircut with someone constantly standing there breathing on the side of their face. You try not to be rude, but they do not understand any hints you have gave them. Eventually you have to tell them, "I'm sorry bro, I have a few people waiting, and I will have to talk to you later." Sometimes you have to let them talk and while you just respond by saying "Um," or nod your head because if you respond with anything more, they will linger and talk for another hour. Come on my peeps; learn how to leave the shop when it's time. Especially know when to leave the barber's area.

FORTY-THREE

The Runner

Let me bring a few Olympic champions back to your remembrance; Carol Lewis, Michael Johnson, Usane Bolt. Any of these names ring a bell? These are some of the fastest runners in the world, but none of them have anything on the customers that run in the barber's chair. Sometimes I wish I could record how they run from the clippers and play it back to them, and maybe they would have a barber's eye view and stop running. I get so tired of chasing lil heads, big heads, and sometimes, huge heads around my chair from day to day that it doesn't make any sense. I can understand chasing a kid around from time to time, but some of these grown men run from the clippers too.

It can get so funny sometime, but it can also become very aggravating to have to chase a grown man from north to south and east to west just to cut his hair. Sometimes I am tempted to not chase them and just leave the haircut just like it is. It seems as if they want you to mess their hair up the way they are always moving their head. If you come to the barbershop to get a haircut, please sit back, sit up, and hold your head still. Your barber will appreciate you, and you will appreciate him for giving you a better haircut because he didn't have to chase you. Stop running; the clippers can't be biting that much!

FORTY-FOUR

The Shop Hopper

I'm sure the majority of us have heard the terminology "church hopper". This is when someone who trying to be religious joins your church, but only stays there until they hear something that they don't like or something was said that uncovered their dirt. This leads them out the door to the next church, only for them to find the same thing there. They leave, and leave, and develop a routine of being unstable. This put them in a worst position than they were when they first started. This is how it is with customers at the barbershop. They find a pretty decent barber, or barbershop, stay there for a while, and out of the blue, you will not see them again until six months down the road. They go somewhere else and get jacked up real bad, and then come running back to you asking if you can fix it. After you fix it, they find another barber the week after, and then another barber the week after. It's almost like playing Russian roulette, only without a gun. You play it with clippers instead. "Let me put this pair on my head and see if I can blow my hairline up!"

People that church hop are like people who will eat off of anyone's table in their neighborhood. Customers that "barber-hop" is not much better because the more barbers you allow playing in your head; the more chances you have at your head getting sick (jacked up, fungus, ringworm). When you find a pretty decent shop, and a pretty decent barber, plant yourself and stop running all over the city. You're not that busy, and you're sure not that important!

FORTY-FIVE

The Last Minute Fade

Although barbering looks like a pretty laid back job, it gets really tiring at times; especially towards the weekend. What most people fail to realize is barbers have to stand on their feet in "ONE" place all day. Of course you know this can get very strenuous on the legs and lower back. Imagine standing on your feet for twelve hours cutting hair, hearing lies, and dealing with crazy customers all day. By this time, your brain is congested, your legs are numb, your back is throbbing, and your knees are gone. It's about time for you to get off and you have your eyes focused on the door because it's the last haircut, so you think. All of a sudden, a customer comes rushing through the door breathing hard and ask, "Man, can you get me real quick?" You think about it briefly, and then respond "Yeah, I got you" In your mind you're thinking why not make a last minute fifteen to twenty dollars. The customer hops in the chair, and decide to get a fade at the last minute of your long day.

Are you serious? It's funny, but I have witnessed some barbers talk some customers out of certain haircuts, especially towards the end of the day. "You sure you want this kind of cut bro?" "You too old for this look." About this time another barber will top off the conversation by saying "Yeah, man, you don't need that cut." It's just like any other team, or army, barbers help each other out whenever possible. All of us know that a last minute fade at the end of the day is crucial, and it's just a "dirty thang" to be requested. Have some sympathy on your barber; don't make his or her day longer than it has already been!

FORTY-SIX

The Sick Man

I f you are a grown man, you have no business going to get a haircut and you know you are sick. What are you thinking to come and sit down in your barber's chair like nothing is wrong with you and spread germs everywhere. There have been times when some customers would almost be about to pass out in the chair while getting a cut because of being sick. Temperature well over a hundred and they still find their way to the barbershop. After you leave the shop, you look better, but you leave all your germs and sickness behind. This put the next man's health in jeopardy, including your barber. It's not like you have other appointments you have to get to. Right after you leave the barbershop, you know you are going home to get in the bed. With this being the case, why can't you just stay in the bed, get over your sickness and then come to get your hair cut. Oh

I forgot, some people are too cool to be in the bed sick with no haircut.

I guess because I'm a barber, I speak for all barbers and hairstylist; we don't want to catch your sickness. We will much rather miss your twenty dollars and stay well to make more, than to get your twenty, get sick and have to take three days off recovering. Taking three days off will cause us to miss hundreds, when we could have only missed your twenty and your cold. Your money is well appreciated, but if you are sick. Please stay home!

FORTY-SEVEN

The Mustache/Goatee Talker

In life, timing is everything. If you are just the slightest off in life, it can cost you everything; including your mustache and goatee. I admit it, it may be a thing in the mind but it seem as if some customers like to talk more at the times they are not suppose to. For example, sometimes you can cut a customer's hair and get total silence during the haircut process. You can take thirty minutes on their hair and they say absolutely nothing, but as soon as you finish the haircut and get to lining up the mustache and goatee, they decide they want to begin talking and laughing. It's almost as if they plan it every time.

I don't know if it's some kind of mental thing for them or what but it seem to happen nine times out of ten. That one customer may understand the importance of not talking when his barber is around his mouth lining his mustache up. I'm grateful for the loyal customers God have blessed me to have, and I'm glad they have confidence in the skill God has blessed me with. At the same time, it doesn't matter how steady your hand is, if the customer is talking and laughing, even the best barber can cut off a mustache. Thank you for trusting your barber, but allow me to speak on his/her behalf. It's better to sit still and be quiet for a couple of minutes and allow him/her to do their job! Stop talking when you are not suppose to and all will be well!

FORTY-EIGHT

The Cheap Man Holding Up the Chair

Attention all barbers. Have you ever had a thirty, forty-dollar customer waiting, but had a cheap, five-dollar customer holding the chair up? You can see your better paying customer is getting impatient and is probably thinking about leaving or letting another barber cut his hair. You are trying your best to get to him but your cheap non-tipping customer keep asking things like, "Can you make sure my line is straight?" or, "Is that the shortest it can go and still be dark?" They find real small things to find just to hold the chair up. Now please allow me to explain myself, every customer is valuable, and important. There are some who just love to make your life miserable, and it seem like they always pick the perfect time to do it. Your ten dollars are just as important as the thirty dollars, but the timing is everything.

FORTY-NINE

The Man Who Disrespects the Freehand

As a barber, you can see just about anything coming. Above all else, you have to respect your old school customers. They will be loyal to you as a customer, even when everyone else will not. The old school guy don't want any trouble, they don't want anything difficult, and they most of the time don't even bother to get a line. I respect the old school, but there is one thing that most old school customers do that gets next to their barber. A lot of them still wear the afro as their desired choice of style, and there is nothing wrong with that. The problem is after your barber have took his, or her time to free hand your afro, comb through it, and free hand it again to get it real good and even, please don't put your hat back on as soon as you get out of their chair. You must understand and respect the art of the free-hand haircut.

It takes a steady hand and a good eye in order to get you back in the game. All we are asking, as your barber is to respect the art, at least until you get back to your car. Most barbers take pride in their work, and to see you place a hat on top of their art is a low blow. I have a couple of old school customers that takes me a good minute to get them back in the game. Some times I feel the sweat running down my back because of the intense concentration. If my name is on it, I want it to look good. The only problem is that old school customers don't care. He is a laid back, easygoing guy and it doesn't matter to him that it took the time it did. As a matter of fact, to him it's not even about the haircut, its just about getting out and about. He is just trying to continue to enjoy life. We love you old school, and we respect you, all we are asking is to get the love back, and the respect for the art of the "free hand."

FIFTY

The Excessive Cologne

'm a firm believer in looking your best, smelling good, and doing well. Let's own up to it, sometimes we can go overboard. I don't know if some customer's nose isn't working, or if they are just immune to the smell of their own cologne, but we have to know when enough is enough. I know we live in a nation that believes in over indulging but we have to train ourselves how to be moderate. There are some customers that sit in your seat and almost burn the hairs, slam out of your nose. It's like they went to the dollar store and bought a bottle of cologne and took the top off and dumped the whole bottle on top of their head just before they came to the barbershop.

If you are a customer, please be advised that you are doing more harm than good when you sit in your barber's chair drenched down with strong cologne. Now don't get me wrong, put on your cologne, look good, smell good, do good, but please don't go overboard. Now and days many are having their own battle with allergies and sinus, and we don't need anything that will be responsible to help trigger it off. Now you got your barber nose running, and he/she can't stop sneezing. All of this plays a part in your finished haircut. If you get out of the chair and feel like you got a terrible cut and it was faster than usual, it may be because of that excessive cologne!

FIFTY-ONE

The Yawner

There is no way in the world you can be so tired that you have to yawn every thirty seconds. Even if you are, try your best to get all of your yawning out before you climb into the barber's chair. It can get real annoying to have to keep watching you stretch your mouth open as wide as you can over and over and over again.

Sometimes I feel like a dentist instead of a barber, because with some customers, I see all their teeth, gums, tonsils and all. What make a barber really frustrated is when you start all that yawning when it's time to get your line. I will admit, I had to push a line or two back because of someone yawning at the wrong time. There is absolutely nothing wrong with yawning, but let's try to get in control, instead of the yawn controlling us. It seems as though some people live to yawn. I guess it makes them feel alive, or give them a sense of satisfaction or something.

I remember I had one young man that yawned so much, I told him he had more yawn (yarn) than Wal-Mart. He didn't understand so I told him he yawned way too much. I started a game with him, and I yawned every time he did. He couldn't do anything but laugh, because we both were yawning every ten to fifteen seconds. He finally began to see himself and was broke out of his yawning habit.

FIFTY-TWO

The Bad Joke Teller

I believe every barbershop has someone that loves to come in and tell a few jokes that they think are hilarious, but they are really terrible jokes. There was a guy that came around maybe once a month to get a cut. While he would wait, he will begin to tell a joke out of the blue. I mean without warning, he would just began to fire them off. At the end of his joke he would be the only one to get it, and he would be almost about to die from laughing. The problem was no one else would get the joke. Everyone else would be laughing, but not at the joke. He thought we were laughing with him, but we were all laughing at him. Oh boy, why did we do that? After he saw that he had the barbershop attention, he would say "Wait, wait, wait, I got another one". There was no shame to his game, and he knew in his mind that he was the greatest at telling jokes. Everyone would say "Naw man, not another one." Little kids would be staring;

all the barbers and customers would be laughing, all prepping ourselves for the next terrible joke. Some people are called to tell jokes around the world, but there are some who are not even called to tell a joke in a place as small as a community barbershop. Check your calling and be sure you have a few really good jokes before you test your skills in public, especially in a public place, such as the barbershop.

FIFTY-THREE

The Angry Man

Have you ever met anyone that's always angry? You really haven't missed anything if you haven't. If you would like too, I give you the invitation to come to the barbershop. There are always a couple of customers that come through the shop that's always mad. One customer in particular came in the shop every two weeks to get a cut. The first few times we didn't think much of it because everyone is entitled to a bad day or two. But this problem kept going on. We finally figured out this was far beyond having a bad day. You can actually feel the angry vibrations pouring out of his head while you were cutting his hair. We all started calling him Murdock because he was always upset!

I remember one day one of the barbers tried to strike a friendly conversation with Murdock, so he asked him, "You enjoying the nice weather?" Murdock replied, "Huh, you should be asking if the weather is enjoying me". From there, every question we would ask Murdock, he will reply with an angry answer. To all angry customers that are out there, I don't know what the world has done to you to make you so upset, but it will help if you tried to smile a while and give your face a rest. It can't possibly be that bad!

FIFTY-FOUR

The Grown Man/Teenage Cry Baby

I believe this is one of the most annoying things to a barber by far. When you get a grown man to sit in your chair and he is constantly running, ducking, and dodging every stroke of the clipper. I don't know if it's because he is that tender headed, or if he is just that fragile. This customer makes me so frustrated, that I felt the frustration while writing this book. It's understandable to chase a small child around the chair, but a grown man; come on dude, man up! I barely touched your head and you're already squeenching your face. Sometimes I wish some of the customer's girl friends would come in and see how fragile their tough acting guy really is. It appears as though some of them need their mother to stand there with them and hold their hand while they are getting a haircut. To every grown man that is still afraid of the clippers, it's time to man up and quit running, what kind of example are you giving to your son and other little leaguers out there?

FIFTY-FIVE

The Man Always Late For His Appointment

I believe every barber have a customer that's always late for their appointment. The reason for setting an appointment is to be there the time you said you would. It's understandable to be late every so often, but I will never understand that customer that's always late. One thing that makes it even worse is when they are late and pull up at the shop; they park and make a phone call like you don't have anyone else to cut. A barber or hair stylist gets frustrated when they have to hear the same excuses about your mishaps on the way to the shop. Do yourself and your barber/stylist a favor; be on time and if you happen to be late, don't stand outside talking on the phone. Time is money in this business.

FIFTY-SIX

The Sleeping Kid

Please understand that it will be a lot easier to cut your child's hair if their head is not bobbing all over the place because they find the barber's chair a bored place and try to take a quick nap in order for time to pass by faster. Every parent I know longs for their child to have a great haircut, and helping see to it that your child is able to hold their head up will play a major part in this outcome. If you want to get in and out of the barbershop as quick as possible, try to allow your child to get rest before he/she gets in the barber's/stylist chair. If you add it all up, hours have been wasted in the shop due to a sleeping child. You wouldn't believe how much faster you can get out of the shop if the barber didn't have to keep stopping due to a sleeping child in the chair.

FIFTY-SEVEN

The Mover

I know there are some people that have uncontrollable twitches but please tell me why you refuse to sit still. Some are kids and believe it or not some are adults that cannot seem to sit still in the seat when they are receiving services. I can slightly understand this problem for a child, but you mean to tell me a grown man finds it hard to be able to concentrate enough to sit still for fifteen minutes. I mean some have to constantly turn, jerk their leg, and mess with the cape, point and everything else while they are getting a haircut. They don't want you to mess up on their haircut but they don't want to sit still. Moving is what they do and they do it well!

I have never seen this problem until I became a barber. It's something about when its time to be still, that's when something in their mind, tells them to move. I know it may be a challenge, but the next time you are in the chair, please sit as still as possible. We don't want you to be a statue or anything but we don't want you moving all over the place either.

FIFTY-EIGHT

The Weak Neck

When you visit your barber/stylist, it is important to be able to keep your neck locked in so that every stroke of the comb, clipper, or brush will not break the neck so to speak. Some times there are customers that seem as though they don't have a bone in their neck. Whenever you cut them against the grain, their head fly backwards like it's about to fly off. When you cut with the grain, their chin is constantly in their chest. It's a no win situation for the barber he/she has to end up holding the customers head up as it is being cut. Maybe the weak-neck customer needs to take some neck vitamins or get calcium shot in the side of their neck. I don't know, but I do know it will help if they can muscle up some strength in their neck at least long enough to get a haircut!

FIFTY-NINE

The Pacer

Man, you're next. Will you please sit down and stop pacing the floor! Pacing is not going to make your barber go any faster. Just as you desire a good haircut, the man that's in the chair deserves one also. Some customers can get so impatient, they will get up, walk around, walk outside, stand by your chair, and everything else they can think of to try to remind you they are there. Sit down, relax and wait until your turn. When you pay attention to time, it seems to go by a lot slower.

SIXTY

The Loud Mouth

Some people just want to be heard and they will make sure they are heard by all means necessary. It seems as though someone that is very loud and outspoken is someone who was overlooked and left out growing up as a child. Now that they are grown, they are making up for all the time they were overlooked. Some customers are loud as soon as they get their foot in the door. From start to finish, the only voice you can hear is their voice! Whether it's a joke, a lie, an invitation, or just a simple conversation, they have to be loud! They are seeking attention and want everyone in the shop to give it to them. If you are loud and know it, save the shop some energy in the atmosphere and lower the tone. It's like everything is zapped out of the atmosphere when they are talking and no one else wants to talk.

SIXTY-ONE

The Man That Know Everything

If it's something I don't like, it's someone who thinks they know everything! It doesn't matter what subject you are discussing, they feel as though they are the only one who know the true answer. There was this one guy who would let everyone talk and share his or her opinions throughout the day. Every single time at the end of each discussion he would say, "This is what it mean." Something would just cringe in me when I would hear him say that. I wanted somebody so bad to ask him why he thinks he know everything. The world is far too big to have just one person in it to have all the correct answers. If you would take the time and be quiet and listen to others, you may learn something for a change. If you are this individual, please stop thinking you know everything because you don't!

SIXTY-TWO

The Man that Throws Out Jokes but Cannot Take Them

The old-school saying is "Don't do the crime if you can't do the time." That's how I feel about telling jokes. There are some people who will come in the shop and have a ball roasting you and enjoy it when they see everyone laughing. They even get the energy to go harder when they get an audience. That's cool, and I have no problem with having a little fun. My problem is when the tables turn and the person that was doing the roasting is now getting roasted and he/she starts getting mad and wants to fight. Everything was alright when they had the crowd going and feeding into their jokes, but they are still having trouble dealing with someone getting the best of them. Grow up my friend, and stop throwing out what you can't take back in!

SIXTY-THREE

The Drooler

There isn't anything more degrading in this world than someone sitting in your chair, falling asleep and drooling all over your chair cloth. Although it's not cool, it's understandable when a small kid drools, but when you are a grown man, you have no business drooling while you are getting a haircut. If you know you are a drooler and you feel yourself falling asleep, it would be to your benefit to start trying to sing, hum, or whistle a song to stay awake. No barber has the time to wash his or her cape off and hang it out to dry because some grown man couldn't keep his mouth closed while he was sleep. Maybe all barbers need to start wearing whistles and blow them really loud when some customers that are known to drool began falling asleep. We're not trying to be funny we just want to be safe. Come and get your haircut but please leave the drool at home!

SIXTY-FOUR

The Kid that wants to See Everything

I love kids, but there are some that need a little bit of TLC. One of my pet peeves with some little kids is their nosiness. There are some kids that I cut on a weekly basis that just want to see everything you reach for. It makes me frustrated when I'm trying to make a move during the haircut and the kid that I'm cutting is following me with his head watching every move I make. I can't even reach for a brush or oil sheen without their little eyes looking and then asking, "What's that for, what's that for, why are you doing that." I understand they learn by asking but I don't understand the nosiness. Every where your hands go, their eyes follow. They watch you throw your trash away, open a piece of gum, count your money and even pick your nose if you had to. Just straight up noisy but you gotta love the kids!

SIXTY-FIVE

The Pop-Up

This may not be something every barber/stylist hate but if you are a barber/stylist that is use to setting appointments with your customers, you hate when someone you have been telling to make an appointment just keep popping up. There are some customers that are just not going to do right if they had to. I have a few customers that know I go mostly by appointments. I have told them over and over to make an appointment with me especially if they are trying to get a cut on the weekend. Every time the say ok, but never follow through. They would rather take their chances and pop up on Friday or Saturday and expect for you to make room for them. You have to realize my friend that the world does not revolve around you. It only takes a few seconds to set an appointment. This would make your world and your barber's world a little simpler. Make an appointment and stop popping up!

SIXTY-SIX

The Blamer

I have learned over the years to scan a customer's head and point out to them any blemishes, spots or bumps that they have prior to the haircut. Some customers love to put the blame on the barber/stylist when they find the slightest thing on their head. Some customers have a bad habit of not washing their hair and have the nerve to blame someone else for the dirtiness and dryness of their scalp. Barbers and stylists are blamed for ringworms, dryness, breakouts, blemishes, bold spots and everything else a customer can think of.

Don't get me wrong, there are some dirty barbers who never clean their clippers or combs and they may be responsible for some of these things but you cant continue to blame them for everything. I guess somebody got to take the blame and be responsible for all of our problems. What you should do is examine your head thoroughly before making your next barbershop visit and you will be surprised at what you find in your head before your barber ever start cutting.

SIXTY-SEVEN

The Staring Kid

Growing up I was taught that it was rude to stare at someone. Staring is something that we all can slip into if we are not careful but there isn't anything that can compare to a kid that stares at you especially around a crowd of people.

In most cases, kids will give you the truth about a matter even if the truth hurts your feelings. Sometimes when a kid is staring at me while I am cutting their hair I can just about count down to the moment they are about to ask an embarrassing question. It seems as though they always pick awkward moments to ask. I've heard kids pick at their barber's teeth, breath, bumps on their face, big lips, big head, and big nose and so on. What makes it even more uncomfortable is that they wait until you spin the chair and they are looking right in your face! "Why your teeth so pointed," you look like Dracula" or "your ears are bigger than Mickey Mouse ears." Of course every one goes to laughing and it urges the kid to keep going. Sometimes the best thing to do is just go along with the game or just walk away for a minute.

SIXTY-EIGHT

The T.V. Watcher

S ome customers will come in, sit in your chair and lock down on the television like a Pit Bull locks down on its victim. Once they lock down they refuse to let go. It's almost like watching the movie poltergeist, only in real life. As the chair turn in one direction, their head turns in the opposite direction to continue watching television.

One time I was cutting a customer and I recognized from the start that I had a TV watcher in the chair but I wanted to see how desperate he was to keep watching. I started spinning the chair very slowly and couldn't believe how he kept his eyes on the show. It felt like the chair almost went completely around before he decided to get with the program and get his haircut finished.

There are some customers that I have now that I just leave the chair in the direction of the television and I walk around the chair instead of spinning it. Nothing can be that important to watch at the risk of breaking your neck.

SIXTY-NINE

The "Get Over" Customer

There are some people in life that are just not going to do right. They strive to beat every system even if it hurt the system they beat. I'm sure if you are a barber or a stylist, you have met the "get over customer" wanting something for nothing! I have experienced for instance customers that sat down and asked how much would it be for a line. I repeat what they said just to be sure we are on the same page. "So all you want is a line right," "yes," they reply, so I said that will be "x" amount of dollars. "Ok that's cool." You give them what they ask for and show them the mirror and they say, "That looks good but can you knock a few of those loose hairs off the top of my head. I said of course but I will have to charge you for a cut. That's when the drama starts. "I thought you said 5-7 dollars how did it jump to 15 dollars. There are far too many mind games out there for people to now try to bring them into the shop. Keep the drama on the outside bro and stop being so cheap trying to get over all of your life! Pay up or get up! Who next?

SEVENTY

The Instigator

You can spot them from a mile away. Yes I'm talking about the instigators. People who love to stick their nose into stuff just long enough to get something started and then they pull out and watch the mess they created unravel.

Every shop have them, you just have to pay very close attention because some of them are not as outspoken as others but they are in the cut somewhere blowing up an issue that was trying to die down.

I remember one guy that use to come to the shop and started an argument or a fight every time he came. As I saw him approaching the shop from the parking lot, my toes began to curl up in my shoes because I knew he couldn't wait to get in to start some mess. Sure enough he would sit down and listen to all the different conversations that were moving through the atmosphere of the shop and like a serpent he would strike in on one that he felt to be most ripe. Argument after argument broke out that he started and then pulled out and enjoyed watching the movie he directed and produced. The sad part is that most people would buy into the garbage that was being directed instead of trying to get the instigator corrected. Some of the same people that laughed this week were his victims the next week. Let's stop the instigator and the instigating and the shop will be a better place.

SEVENTY-ONE

The Tender Head

What can you do? You can't brush it, you can't comb it, you can't wash it, and you can barely cut it! I'm glad I haven't met many but there are some customers that I have taken far too long on because of them having a tender head. I wish that they will pre-comb, brush and/or wash their hair before they even think about taking a step toward the shop. You see them jumping and jerking, dodging and crying because their scalp is over sensitive to everything that comes in contact with it. I wouldn't doubt if they didn't say "ouch" when the sunlight hit their head. I feel sorry for them because they really can't sit back and enjoy the true pleasure it is to come to the shop/salon. A haircut and a shampoo is one of the most relaxing things a person can ever experience unless you are tender-headed. The stylist can't massage your head and the barber has to be careful while cutting your head. Man, you really don't know that you are missing the full benefits of your trip to see your barber/stylist.

SEVENTY-TWO

The Tickled Kid

Cutting a kids hair can be an advantage or a BIG disadvantage. My cousin cuts hair in Wilmington, N.C. He once told me that he cut some people so fast that he would feel bad when taking their money. This is how it is suppose to be with kids. I mean, their head is small and round and it seems as though you can cut one in about 5 minutes, ten at most. The only problem is, sometimes you get that kid that is very ticklish and jumps and laugh every time you attempt to cut.

I have witnessed one little ticklish kid hold up the chair for over thirty minutes. It's cute for the first thirty seconds but it gets old after that. It really gets old fast if you have five or six other customers already backed up waiting on you. Usually it's mom that brings the kid and she is just standing there laughing at her son/daughter holding up the chair. Please understand that time is money, especially in the shop! We don't care about the kids laughing but we do care about how long. If we are not careful a small ticklish problem can get out of hand really quickly. So hold your head down so I can get the back of your neck and stop all that laughing.

SEVENTY-THREE

The Destructive Child

Are you serious? You mean to tell me you are just going to stand there and watch your child try to destroy the shop. I'm sorry, but some kids are more destructive than an atomic bomb and I refuse to let them be that way in this shop! Everywhere they go they have to touch something. They pull on the chair while they are getting a cut. They pull on the clipper cords. Not to mention that they try to tear a hole in the chair cloth. I have watched them knock down all the greenery, while messing up the magazines on the table. The list goes on and on. The question is when are the parents of these kids going to step in and do something. I'll tell you what; we are going to start charging extra due to the level of destructiveness of the child. Although I'm just kidding, it sure sounds good because there are some children, which act as though they have absolutely no training at home. It's sad to say, but some of them do not. A public embarrassment is only the result of poor private training. Let's get control of our children and keep them from costing us everywhere we take them.

SEVENTY-FOUR

The No Neck

It's hard enough trying to cut someone that refuses to lift there head in order for you to cut the hair under their neck but it's even more frustrating to cut someone that has no neck at all. Every now and then you will get a customer to sit in your chair that you want have to worry about pulling the chair cloth down trying to get around their neck. This customer may seem simple but it's a struggle trying to give them a line or a shave. It almost seems as if they are purposely trying to shrink their neck down to give you a hard time. I have to pump my chair up as high as it could go in order to complete the haircut. It seem as though their head is just sitting on their shoulders.

SEVENTY-FIVE

The Man that Think He knows what He is Talking about but have no Idea

It is hilarious to see someone walk in the shop and try to talk like a barber when he or she is explaining what kind of haircut he or she wants. I remember a fellow walked into the shop trying to look all-important. His turn finally came around to get a cut and he said with confidence "give me a 0.5 millimeter against the grain" the shop went silent for about a tenth of a second and burst out with laughs from everywhere. You could tell he didn't know what he as talking about because he had dark wavy hair. We tried to tell him that he was about to have a baldhead but he tried to hold on to what he thought he knew. The debate went on for a few minutes and he finally gave in. We asked him if he wanted to keep it dark and he said yeah. "Boy, I'm glad I didn't give you what you asked for because we probably would've been fighting when you looked in the mirror." To make a long story short, he ended up getting a two against the grain. Still dark, still wavy, and everybody was able to still be happy.

SEVENTY-SIX

The Gas Expresser

Come on man! You didn't have to eat what you know gives you an upset stomach right before you sit in my chair every time do you? All the years that we spend with ourselves, we yet neglect to learn anything about ourselves. If you know that every time you eat a certain food that doesn't agree with your stomach, you should have enough sense not to eat that food before coming to the shop. Nothing is unhealthier than inhaling someone else stomach problems.

Some people just don't care what they do to themselves or to each other. I had a customer one time that kept making funny faces and squirming in the chair. I didn't think anything of it at first but when he continued to do it, immediately I knew what the deal was. I started from that moment on cutting his hair as fast as I could because I knew if I didn't, we were going to have problems real soon. As soon as I finished, he ran out the door and I never saw him in the shop again. I respect him though for holding it in instead of letting it all go! Thanks bro.

SEVENTY-SEVEN

The Slumpper

Out of everything you may have to teach a customer, how to sit up in the chair shouldn't be one of them. It really gets under a barber/stylist's skin when we have to constantly ask a customer to please sit up. One of the sad parts about it is, most of the time it's the same customer. "Didn't we just go over this last week?" if you are reading this and you are someone that jumps in the chair and don't know how to sit up, after reading this, please make it less stressful for your barber or stylist and sit up in the chair. Here you are making something that should be a 10 or 15-minute job turn into something a whole lot longer because you want to be cool, or stubborn. Slumping is not made for any chair, and it's definitely not made for a barber's chair.

SEVENTY-EIGHT

The Gum Chewer

Chewing gum is an American tradition that most people have adopted as a habit. I have no problem with chewing gum because I chew it myself. The problem I have is *"when"* the gum is being chewed. During a haircut gum chewing really doesn't play a factor, but I don't understand why some customers have to chew it when they are getting a line after the cut. In some cases it's some of the pickiest customers that don't want their line crooked, or their taper jacked up that pick the wrong time to start chewing their gum like its going out of style. It seem as though they would have enough sense to realize that the barber can better serve them without any extra distractions coming from them.

If you have an overwhelming urge to chew your gum during your shape up or taper, just ask if you can toss it out and watch how quick your barber/stylist give you the trash can. Gum is fine but it's even better when you chew it at the right time! Your barber/stylist is on your side and they want to always give you the best service. You deny them that right when you hop in their chair chewing gum and blowing bubbles. The gum can wait and you will be the beneficiary of a good haircut.

SEVENTY-NINE

The "Am I next" man

Ok, so you just walked in the shop and see that it is beyond packed out. Customers standing around the wall and you automatically ask are you next? Going even further, you keep asking after each person gets up out of the chair. The best thing you can do is make an appointment, or ask your barber how many do he/she have in front of you. The trick is to ask them "ONE TIME" and then sit down.

The last time I checked, the world didn't revolve around one customer and I don't think it's going to start today. You may be cool, you may have swag, and you may even have a little bit of paper, but you have to wait in line just like everyone else. When your time come around trust me the finger will be pointed at you and you want have to ask another time "am I next?"

EIGHTY

The Appointment Canceller

Attention all customers! The sole purpose for setting an appointment is to make it to the appointment. I don't have a clue why some people set appointments but never make them. It must make them feel bubbly inside or just important to be able to call you and say put me down for such-and-such time. I like customers that make appointments but I love customers who actually make them. There are some that set appointments faithfully and never show up faithfully. Sometimes if they show up they are thirty to forty minutes late and still expect for you to squeeze them in. If you are not able to fit them in, they think you are doing them wrong but they can never see that they have done you wrong all year by cancelling 90% of their appointments they made with you throughout the years. If you know you are one that cannot keep an appointment, just don't make one. Be a walk-in and life will be better for you and your barber/stylist.

EIGHTY-ONE

The man that doesn't know what he wants but expects you to know

've had customers who had no clue what they want and they try to explain a style that is floating around in their head but never do a good job at explaining. When their barber/stylist gets the puzzled face, the customer gets offended and tries to make the barber feel less than a barber for not being able to read his/her mind. If you can't properly explain your haircut don't expect for anyone else to be able to. In most cases, the style they are thinking about is for people with hair. Please try not to go off the deep-end when your barber/stylist have no clue to the image or make-believe thought you have floating around in your head. If you can't see it, it's going to be hard for anyone else to see it.

EIGHTY-TWO

The Drunk Man

Cutting a drunk man/woman is not fun. Number one; before you finish, it's going to feel like you are drunk due to the scent that you will experience throughout the haircut. Number two; you never know what a drunk person is thinking. I've seen them go off, cuss, hallow, fall out, and even start fights. They can't keep their head up, they sweat constantly, and sometimes they act as though they don't understand when you start talking about price.

It's funny, but I've had the opportunity to witness a drunk man empty out his pockets to a barber and told him to keep the change. I don't know how much it was but it was well more than the cost of a haircut. I don't think he would've given him that much if he wasn't drunk. I guess cutting a drunk man's hair sometimes goes in a barber's favor and sometimes it goes against him/her. Either way I prefer the man minus the alcohol. Sober up, sit up, and pay up!

EIGHTY-THREE

The B.O.

I know that there is no way in the world you are not able to detect that you are in code red with your B.O. Sometimes I wonder why a person's spouse, friend, mother, father or what have you, will not tell the person they say they love that they are ranking. No one can be that immune! Some say they have become immune to their own bad breath and body odor but there has to be someone brave enough to pull you to the side to tell you to try to clean yourself up a little. Especially before you go to the barbershop.

The shop can get crowded and hot, on top of the cape that has to go on top of you prior to your haircut. We all know what happens when a bunch of people gather together and get to talking and lying. Things heat up real fast and scents that could be covered in the cold are exposed in the heat! I understand that some people must shower two to three times a day. If that's you, try to come to the shop directly after you have showered. Your barber/ stylist will thank you for it!

EIGHTY-FOUR

The Parent that stands next to you watching your every move

There's nothing worse than someone telling you how to do something they don't know how to do themselves. There are some parents that will hover over your small workspace trying to play good parent and coach at the same time. First of all, a barber's space is already tight and you mean to tell me you are going to make it tighter! I don't understand how someone who doesn't know the first thing about cutting hair could stand in your way and tell you how to do your job. Mechanics know cars, accountants know numbers, architects know buildings, and barbers know hair.

It really bothers me to see a parent standing over their kid's barber/stylist watching every stroke of the clipper and every clipping of the scissors. They stand there pointing, looking and demanding you to do things that you already planned to do. They want correct their child when they see them cutting up but they sure will correct you when they assume that you are making the wrong move with the clippers.

It gets really sad when a mother feels as though she have to stand beside her teenage son, or stand there and tells her forty-year-old husband how he should get his haircut. Back up, give the barber his/her space and correct what you don't like after the cut is over.

EIGHTY-FIVE

The Pouting Kid

Although pouting takes a lot of energy, there are several kids that are determined to pout every trip to the barbershop. It seems as though they would grow into the experience and get comfortable with getting a haircut but there are some kids who refuse to make your job easy from day to day. They throw themselves in your chair, fold their arms and stick out their lips to let you know they are angry. I have grown numb to it now and just ignore it and get the haircut over with as fast as I can.

There is one kid I cut on a weekly basis that acts like a little baby every week. His routine never fails. He comes through the door pouting, sit in the chair pouting, and leave out pouting. Please teach your kids how to assist in making their haircutting experience more pleasurable by trying to smile instead of pout. It makes me want to take off my belt and give them a good old fashion spanking. Maybe that is what's missing in the equation. When we spare the rod, we spoil the child. There has been too much rod sparring and we are left with far too many spoiled, unthankful children. Unfold your arms, smile and sit up in this chair so we can do our job!

EIGHTY-SIX

The Impatient kid

Going on a trip with a child can be a two-edged sword. On the trip, you are bound to experience excitement and frustration. You never know which one you will get and when you will get it. If you don't have any babysitting tools such as games, movies, toys, etc., you are bound to hear the million dollar question a million times; "Are we there yet?" The down side to this impatience is that it follows a child everywhere they go, including the barbershop.

A barber/stylist has to reach deep down within to overcome the constant question "Are you done yet?" This echoes through the voice of an impatient kid that occupies their chair. Truth be told, the barber or stylist is really more concerned about being finished than the child. There isn't anything like a bad, impatient kid sitting in your chair holding you up from doing your job. If you hear your child constantly asking, "are you done yet," chances are he/she has a frustrated barber. Please keep in mind, a frustrated barber is not the kind of barber you want cutting your child's hair. It would help if you step in and calm your child down so they can receive the best haircut ever!

EIGHTY-SEVEN

The Two-Year Old Line-Up

I understand that everyone wants to see their child look the cutest after stepping down out of the barber's chair but there are some things that are pushing it. There are parents that know their child doesn't like to get a haircut and he sure don't like holding his head still to put a line on it.

Even after the parent witness the barber struggles and efforts to cut their child's hair, the parent still insist that their two year old get a line put on their head. Every two year old is not going to sit still long enough to get a line after their haircut and we have to come to reality with this. We shouldn't get mad with the barber if we can't control our child to sit still while the barber is trying his/her best to cut the child's hair. Putting a line on a two- year old kid that refuses to sit still is a lot harder than it appear. Help your barber help you. Hold your child still or stop requesting the styles that require stillness!

EIGHTY-EIGHT

The Trash-Talker

Have you ever met somebody and all they do is talk trash? I mean every time you see them they got something crazy, or negative to say. They talk trash about sports, trash about politics, and trash about their job, and everything else they come in contact with. I have met many of these characters for the first time in the barbershop. They come in and scan the room to scope out the conversation or person they can start talking trash about. Trust me, it never takes them long.

I know a few of them that I can count down before they began talking trash. Sometimes I just want to tell them, "Man, all you do is talk trash," but I save myself the drama because it will only stir up something that may get ugly really fast! I have just learned over the years that some people are so miserable; the only satisfaction they get throughout the day is trying to make someone else miserable. Hopefully one day they will come to grips with life and get delivered from the trash they carry within.

EIGHTY-NINE

The Hater

You haven't seen a hater until you have seen one in the barbershop. Some guys just want all the attention, and if they see someone else getting a compliment, or attention, the hating begins.

As a barber, I sit back and examine the rest of the game and have fun laughing at 40 year old men still hating on each other. It should come to a point in our lives where we give up trying to be cool, or best dressed. Let the young boys have the game of hating. Sometimes I have witnessed grown men hating on each other so bad that arguments and fights got started. The hating really begins when a woman is in the mist of the shop with a lot of men. Some men can't handle a woman complimenting another man, so before she compliment on something, the hater already go on attack mode and try to minimize a new pair of shoes or a nice outfit the other guy has on. It doesn't pay to hate. It seem as though some people were born hating. Get the hating out your heart and you probably will live longer.

NINETY

The Sudden Jumper

Cutting hair is an art. With this being the case, those that are receiving a haircut have to learn how to respect the art. Imagine you sitting next to one of the greatest artist of all-time while he/she was in the process of painting a priceless masterpiece. All of a sudden without warning you jumped and bumped their arm as they were adding the finishing touches to make it that priceless original. Oops will not fix this! This is an illustration to show you how a sudden jumper in their chair can distract a barber. You can be focused on finishing up a cut and all of a sudden the customer jumps without given any warning. They can jump from being ticklish, a sudden chill, or the clipper grabbing them or maybe something else. Whatever they jump for, I wish I could know that it's coming.

I have been blessed thus far to be able to pull the clippers away real fast before any damage that is beyond fixing is done. Most jumpers are kids, but I have cut some teens and sad to say some adults that jump as well. If you feel as though you have to jump, try to warn your barber or stylist or pray they have a quick reflex to pull the clippers back.

NINETY-ONE
The Exaggerator

Many people get their fulfillment by bringing others into their imaginary life they are living inside of their head. I have never seen people that exaggerate like I witness in the barbershop. I never understood why people have to stretch what's already true. All of us are guilty of exaggerating at times in our life but I can't understand the person that makes a living out of stretching everything.

If you go fishing and catch ten fish, don't come in the shop bragging about how you caught a cooler full of fish. Or, if you met a lady that look fairly decent, don't go around telling people your girlfriend remind you of Janet Jackson or Gabriel Union. I guess people feel like when they exaggerate it makes them look better or bigger. Truth be told, it really makes them look smaller once the real truth comes out.

I don't know why people feel like they have to exaggerate when they come into the barbershop but this is the place where exaggerating was born. In most cases it's men that feel like they have to stretch the truth in order to be accepted but I have meet some women also that have this habit of making things seem better than what they really are. As a barber/stylist, we have to sit back and listen to this foolishness constantly and it's time that I tell you the truth; you don't have to lie, just tell it like it *"tis."*

NINETY-TWO

The Acting Child

Nine times out of ten, every barber or stylist has a child that gets up in the chair and act like you are killing them. They jump, and move at every little thing you do. They cry, yell, and pout at the slightest touch of the clipper or comb. You know that you are not hurting them but their acting skills seem to even fool you at times. You stop cutting, or combing only to find out they were just putting on. Sometimes I think about getting a charter bus and finding every child that loves to act out in the barber chair and drop them off in Hollywood. I'm telling you, Hollywood can discover the next great actor if they made a trip to the barbershop.

I had a kid that I was cutting that was jumping and crying through the entire haircut. Every time I touched him, he would say "that hurt." Finally I got frustrated and wanted to see if he was really serious. I left the clipper running and act like I was still cutting but I wasn't touching his head at all. As I was acting as though I was cutting, I asked him, "does that hurt," he said "yes." At that point I knew I had an actor in the chair. I told him that I didn't even touch him that time. After he knew I was on to him he started laughing and straightened up from there after.

NINETY-THREE

The Eye Staring

The eyes are said to be one of the gateways to the soul. With this being the case, there are some people that you rather not stare into your soul. I understand a child looking into your eyes and trying to figure out who you are, but to have a grown man staring into another grown man's eyes is just uncaused for. There are a few customers that you can see staring into your eyes as you are cutting their hair. It's like they don't have anything else to focus on throughout the entire barbershop but into your eyes. I get it sometimes while I am giving a customer a line-up. You're talking about the most uncomfortable feeling in the world when you realize a grown man is staring you down. This is something a barber really doesn't like so please stop doing it. The only eyes a man should gaze into on that note are his wife eyes. When this happens I have learned to spin the chair and work on something else. You want your barber or stylist to be as comfortable as possible so try not to do the stare thing or anything else to throw off their comfort zone. Remember, you deserve the best haircut and something may go wrong if your barber/ stylist is uncomfortable.

As a child my mother taught me it was disrespectful to stare at someone. It can say a lot to the person that is being stared at i.e., you're weird, something is in your nose, something is wrong with you, etc. To save a person the thought of something being wrong with them just try not to look at them for a long length of time. Always remember if something is done to you that make you feel uncomfortable, try not to do it to anyone else.

NINETY-FOUR

The Misbehaved Child

Your child misbehaves badly and you are fully aware of it. If you know it, so why aren't you doing anything about it? There isn't anything like a child that is acting up and the parent isn't doing anything about it. I've witnessed kids in my chair doing everything possible other than sitting still. From start to finish they are acting like Bae-Bae kids. They pull on all the cords, jump in the chair, and grab the comb and brush and everything else you could imagine. Sometimes they ask you embarrassing questions and even pass gas in your chair. Trust me, you run across some bad kids in the barbershop. I had one kid that pulled the neck strip off his neck, pulled the chair cloth over his head, and begin screaming, refusing to get a haircut. In those times I often think if I chose the right profession.

NINETY-FIVE

The Caller

I'm sure every barber/stylist has a customer that constantly calls. "How many you got?" sometimes the reason they call is so unnecessary and untimely. It's quit all right to call your barber but not everyday. It can get annoying real quick to have a grown man constantly calling you asking about a haircut and other things that are so irrelevant.

I have had customers call me that were an hour and a half away from the shop asking me how many people I had, or was anybody in the chair. Being that you are so far away, regardless if anyone was in the chair or not, about time you get here I'm sure a few people will be ahead of you. I don't know the reason for these unnecessary calls but they can get old real fast. Save yourself some cell phone minutes and stop calling people so much. You may have a real emergency that you will be thankful about non-important calls that you made to worry your barber/stylist.

NINETY-SIX

The Shop Pleaser

There are some people that really fight for attention. These people are so unfulfilled; they will try to please a crowd by all means necessary. There have been brothers that came in the shop trying to be comedians, rappers, fix-it men, and so on. It seem as though these people always wait until the shop gets full and then begin to brag. Whatever they felt like they had to do in order to gain a friend or get a few brownie points, that's what they did. You can tell these people don't get much attention at home or anywhere else so they feel like they will try the barbershop.

When I'm cutting hair and recognize someone is trying to please everybody in the shop it really gets under my skin. Most of the time the joke is not funny and the rapping they are trying to do is making no sense at all. I really feel sorry for them and wish they really found a comfortable place in life where they can just be themselves. If you are reading this, I want to assure you that you don't have anyone to try to please but God. Save yourself the effort and the strength my friend.

NINETY-SEVEN

The "Nodder"

I tell everyone, there isn't anything like a nap in the barber's chair. Just the experience of closing your eyes, hearing the buzzing of the clippers, and feeling the warmth of the blade moving back and forth across your head. The only thing is you must be a professional while you are napping so that you will not slow the barber down with a bunch of nodding. What I mean by a professional is that some people can sleep and continue to keep their head held upright and the barber never has to miss a beat.

On the contrary, there are some customers that have a habit of nodding to the point of extreme. It seems as if they pick the wrong times to nod. Just when you are getting ready to shape-up their front line, or when you are trying to tighten up the goatee. Sometimes when you are putting the finishing touches on a tight fade, they pick that time to start nodding off on you. If it weren't for the ability to jerk the clippers away from the customer's head, many customer's haircuts would be messed up due to nodding. If you are not a professional sleeper, please be well rested before your next barbershop visit.

NINETY-EIGHT

The "can you fix this" man

Some customers will come to you faithfully for weeks and all of a sudden they get missing. After awhile they will show back up complaining about how another barber messed their hairline up or their haircut period! I believe once you find something you like, stick with it. Regardless of what I like, there are people who would rather go from barber to barber complaining about how the last barber did them wrong.

It's almost like church. People go from church to church and have something negative to say about each one they visit. I have also known some customers try to do a quick fix on their own head and something went terribly wrong! Of course they always would come running back to you begging you to save their appearance for the weekend. Sometimes you can fix it, and sometimes it's beyond repair. The best thing to do is to leave your head alone and allow the professionals to do their job! Find a good barber/stylist and stick with him/her.

NINETY-NINE

The man that need to see the mirror before each haircut

I may be wrong, but I thought you live with yourself everyday. If you live with yourself everyday, chances are you have to see yourself everyday. In other words you shouldn't be so quick to forget what you look like. I'm sure when you washed your face this morning and knew you were on your way to the barbershop, you saw what the hair on your head and face looked like. It would be a good idea to already have in mind what kind of cut you would like, and what you want to do with your face.

Nevertheless there are guys that come in faithfully every week and ask for the mirror when they sit down in the chair. It's like clock work. A clock does the same thing all the time. I have gotten into a habit of handing them the mirror before they ask for it now. When this happen they look at me like I'm a mind reader or something. Far be it from the truth.

I just know the routine of all of my customers now and the mirror thing is something that's funny but yet annoying at the same time. Know your face; know your cut, save some time. Someone else is waiting in line for a cut behind you.

ONE HUNDRED

The Man that Always ask, "How Much DO I Owe You"

For the most part, the price of haircuts doesn't fluctuate in price every month. Yet and still, you have that faithful customer that get out of your chair and ask, "How much do I owe you?" this can become very annoying to a barber. Trust me, if there is a price change, you as the customers will be the first to know. Without you (the customer) there is no us (the barber). Thank you for your consideration of wanting to pay us correctly but if you are a dollar short, we will let it be known. It's nothing you have to stop asking, but if you want to save yourself the breath, just pay and don't ask the amount. Once again, if the price does change, you will be advised!

ONE HUNDRED ONE
The "Dap-it-Up" Man

I f we are not careful, we can become too excessive in the slightest things in life and not even know it. Have you ever taken the time to think if you had a habit that maybe wasn't a big deal to you? Sometimes what's not a big deal to you could be very bothersome to someone else. I don't have a problem at all with customers that give me dap. The problem I have is how they do it, and of course how many times.

We had a customer that came in the shop and gave everybody in the shop some dap. Every barber and customer, rather he knew you or not. When he came in and when he was leaving out. It was like an announcer calling out the starting line-up and he was the point-guard or something that runs out and dap-up the team and the fans. Dap is good, but too many is ridiculous! I also have a problem with thirty and forty year old men trying to still be cool and have a handshake that takes thirty minutes to complete. They take you through all these different movements. It's funny because it seem as though they lose themselves in the handshake by trying to be so cool. One dap and a regular handshake is acceptable for the day. Your barber will appreciate you sparing them the risk of wrist failure.

WHAT DOES YOUR GROOMING SAY ABOUT YOU?

Nothing boosts your confidence more than being well groomed. Grooming says to the next man/woman how much you think of yourself. What does your grooming say about you? Your self-worth, value, and esteem can sometimes be determined by how others see you invest in yourself. Sure, it can seem time consuming in the upkeep of yourself but it's always well worth it. Think about it; how many more times will there be another you? The answer is never. With this being the case, why not aim your best with the one shot that you are allowed.

The small things such as a shower, haircut, dressing nice, as well as smelling nice are all known to build your esteem to heights beyond your wildest dreams. Studies show that we are more effective and motivated when we are well groomed. Nothing compares to the feeling of waking up and showering first thing in the morning. Wash your face, practice good hygiene, comb/brush your hair and everything else in between that's necessary for the greater you!

Have you ever been on the bad side of grooming? Another way of saying this is, have you ever lost any opportunity or was treated differently because of poor grooming? You could be in the dark to the fact of not getting the job you interviewed for, or not being called for that second date, or maybe even that kiss good night. All of this and more can possibly be linked to poor personal grooming. Let's be honest, I haven't met anyone that loves to smell bad breath or B.O. Try hard to not be the one that is talked about concerning poor grooming.

In most cases you will be primarily remembered for your grooming and attire. You can call it judging or stereotyping but that doesn't stop reality from being reality. People will always be people and there are many that will study your grooming habits in order to make a decision about you. Appropriate grooming supports your image and let others know that you are a person which takes a lot of thought about yourself. Good grooming also speaks a lot about a man or woman's personality. Let your personality speak well for you by the way you keep yourself groomed. Always remember you are well worth looking good and feeling good!

GROOMING TIPS FOR MEN

- **Hair**

  For a more even and precise cut, thoroughly shampoo and dry your hair before a trip to your local barber/hair stylist. This will allow your hair to be free from grease, oils, dirt etc. your scalp will be able to freely breathe therefore causing your hair to stand correctly for a more even haircut throughout.

  If you are planning to get a bald cut, this technique will greatly benefit you as well as allow you to experience a smoother bald head. Again, shampoo your hair and make sure that your scalp is "squeaky clean." If you have a very low cut or fizzies growing back from a previous bald cut, it may benefit you to place a hot steamed towel on your head for maybe 15-30 seconds. This cleans and opens up pores so that the razor can cut even closer than usual.

If you're going in to just get an edge-up/line-up, clean thoroughly around the hairline with an antiseptic on some form of cotton swab. The skin is free from dirt and excess oils therefore leaving a more crisp line/edge. This technique also works best for a razor line as well.

- **Face**

Sometimes facial blemishes are responsible for causing many distractions. These blemishes may cause the person that has them to be self-conscious about his or her appearance, therefore causing them not to perform well are think clearly. These so-called imperfections may also distract others that are engaging in conversation with you. Their eyes are constantly drawn to the pimple(s) or blemishes as they are talking to you. They are distracted, you are uncomfortable due to their deep stare and the conversation doesn't reach its peak in which it was attended to.

Lightly dampen face with warm to hot water. Afterwards cleanse face with a facial cleanser of your preference. There are countless facial cleansers that are on the market that are credible. Do some researching until you find the facial cleansing line of products that work best for you. It would help to know if you have normal, oily, or dry skin. Your cleanser will be based upon your skin type. After the cleanser, you will benefit by an exfoliator or a cleansing mask. You can't go wrong either way you decide to go. Thoroughly cleanse the excess exfoliator or mask off and follow up with a good toner and daily moisturizer.

- **Chapped lips**

   Chapped or dry lips are a common problem amongst thousands of people. Chapped and cracking lips can be very unattractive. Keep those lips under control by adding the right amount of chap-stick throughout the day. Cracked and dry lips are a sure confidence buster.

- **Smell nice**

   After a hot shower, spray on a body fragrance of your choice. Be careful not to overdo it. Too much is a turn-off even if it's a great fragrance. Try to spray on fragrances until you find the one that best flows with your body chemistry.

- **Clean hands/Nails**

  Women notice and love nice clean hands. Wash your hands frequently and clean your nails regularly to make sure that they don't have any dirt stuck in them. Dirty hands and nails are a sure turn off. Dry rough hands are not attractive either. A good hand lotion can work miracles if consistently used.

- **Practice good posture**

  Stand tall and walk without a slump. Slumping is a sign of lacking confidence. Standing and sitting are the same. The way someone sits speaks a lot about that person. Good posture increases our thinking ability by allowing more oxygen to the brain. As our brain receives more oxygen we are able to think more. People with good postures are said to be more attractive. Someone with a good posture carries themselves in a more confident way.

- **Dress nice**

  Dressing well doesn't necessarily mean you have to spend a lot of money. Wear clothes that fit. Clean clothes will help. Never be afraid to wear colors that compliment your personality. (You like what you like). When in doubt you can always ask a friend or either hire an image consultant to help with your wardrobe. Social media has literally thousands of sights that may assist you with putting colors and patterns together. Dressing nice is a instant confidence booster.

- **Water**

    Water causes all parts of the body to function correctly. When the body is functioning at its highest peak, the happier you will be and the better you will feel. Simply put water can put you in a better mood. Many positive benefits comes from drinking water i.e., increased energy, weight loss, less headaches due to less toxins in the body, complexion improved due to moisturizing the skin and many more. Try to remain hydrated.

- **Rest**

    Everyone should try to get a proper amount of sleep. Sleep helps keep your mind and body healthy, energized, and alert. A lack of sleep will make you feel moody and inadequate. Many things can come in between you and a good nights rest. Things such as stress on the job, financial obligations, family challenges and so on. You may not be at fault of none of the before mentioned however, you can build a routine that may lead to better rest i.e. not eating or drinking after a certain time at night, not going to bed at different hours of the night, turning the television off instead of watching it thinking it will cause you to fall asleep faster.

- **Exercise**

Feeling better, living longer, being more positive, is all connected to exercising regularly. Look no further than exercise. The health benefits of regular exercise and physical activity are hard to ignore. There are countless benefits when it comes to exercising. Exercise is known to control your weight, help with health issues, boosts energy and stamina as well as help better mood swings. A lack of grooming has a lot to do with a low mood or feeling depressed. Exercise can help this altogether.

GROOMING TIPS
FOR WOMEN

- **Hair**

   Managing your hair by changing your hairstyle from time-to-time will boost your confidence quickly. Being loyal to your stylist is very important. They have the "411" on your hair and have grown prone to know the hair styles that will fit best for your face. They will tell you pony tails are cute however they shouldn't be worn every day. Try washing your hair two to three times a week followed by a good conditioner. Avoid digging into your hair with foreign objects i.e., bobby pins, paper clips, the tips of scissors, etc., this could cause scratches and bruises that could lead to scalp irritation when chemicals are added.

- **Remove the excess**

   Removing excessive hair will be very

enhancing. Hair around the lips is very unattractive for women. Try to free this area from all hair growth at all times. Eye brows should be attended to and shaped at least once in four to five weeks. Hair from your legs, arms, underarms, etc should be removed when possible. If you're trying to be elegant and classy it's very unattractive to be known as a "hairy" woman.

- **Hands and feet (Finger nails and toe nails)**

  Dirty fingernails are a turn-off to men not to mention the harm to health. Aim for the classy looking nail and maintain a manicure the French manicure. Manicures are known to keep the nails looking clean, neat and healthy.

  Keep your toe nails clipped and well trimmed. Overgrown rugged toenails can damage your self-image in the eyes of others. Rough feet are not preferred by neither gender, but females should definitely seek to keep soft smooth feet. Pedicures periodically will be a great choice to smooth those rough edges and keep those feet looking and feeling silky.

- **Even your facial skin tone**

  Make-Up can give you a smooth complexion

and a glowing appearance. After choosing a facial makeup of your preference, smooth out your face and cover up all known blemishes. An even skin tone on your face is very attractive.

- **Lip liner**

    A lip liner is recommended for that 3Dimesional look that is a sure esteem booster. Using a lip liner enhances the way your lips look. They can make the lips appear to be smaller or larger, depending on color and how you apply it. Lip liners are available in countless colors. Pick your shade according to the look you're pursuing. Before you apply your lipstick try to outline your lips with a lip liner first and watch the magic!

- **Perfume**

    A light perfume will always brighten up your day as well as those around you. Remember not to overdo it. At the end of the day you want to attract instead of repel. Perfume is known for boosting your mood. When you smell good, you feel good about yourself. Spray on a few sprays of your favorite perfume and watch its benefits. It is capable of relieving your stress freeing your mind, and making you feel like a million bucks.

ABOUT THE AUTHOR

Ronald Wilson was born in Wilmington, North Carolina. He and his wife Rachel were called into the ministry and ordained pastors by the late Bishop John W. Barber in 1998. Wilson is the author of *The Dream Team*. An inspiring writing concerning those whom God chooses to walk with you while on your road to destiny. *The Dream Team* was blessed to receive a foreword by Bishop Michael A. Blue, author of Building Credibility in Leadership and founding pastor of The Door of Hope Christian Church in Marion, South Carolina.

He and his wife Rachel are both licensed Life Coaches with credentials from Saint Thomas Christian University in Jacksonville, Florida. Wilson and his wife Rachel both received honorary doctorate degrees from Saint Thomas as well. They are currently the Senior Pastors of Kingdom Vision Life Center in Greensboro, North Carolina.

CONTACT THE AUTHOR

Ronald Wilson
2705B West Gate City Blvd.
Greensboro, North Carolina 27403

336-850-1044
336-609-2127

www.kvlcgso.gmail.com

**Additional resources by Ronald Wilson
are available i.e., DVDs CDs
Please contact Kingdom Vision Media Ministry
2705 B West Gate City Blvd.
Greensboro, N.C. 27403
336-850-1044
336.609.2127
www.kvlcgso@gmail.com**

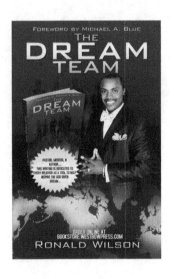

Pick up your copy of **The Dream Team**
today by visiting online @ **BOOKSTORE.
WESTBOWPRESS.COM**